Developing communication and counselling skills in medicine

...s is now widely recognized. ...ery from illness, decreasing ...reducing common causes of ...rse and *Developing communi-* ...th a predominantly practical

...sionals on how to deal with ...how the reader can acquire ...of case examples. As well as ...h, there are chapters dealing ...s find themselves – breaking ...d, or interviewing angry or ...importance of a self-support ...h can offer further help to ...nicians with extensive know-

...Psychiatry, London. She also ...holomew's Hospital, London and at the Centre for Health Studies, University of Kent at Canterbury.

The contributors: Russell Blacker, James Calnan, Anthony Clare, Jeremy Coid, Linda Gask, Roger Higgs, Nira Kfir, Janice Kohner, Peter Maguire, Robert Newell, Maurice Slevin, Averil Stedeford, Jenifer Wilson-Barnett.

Developing communication and counselling skills in medicine

Edited by
Roslyn Corney

Tavistock/Routledge
London and New York

First published in 1991
by Routledge
11 New Fetter Lane, London EC4P 4EE

Simultaneously published in the USA and Canada
by Routledge
a division of Routledge, Chapman and Hall Inc.
29 West 35th Street, New York, NY 10001

Typeset by Leaper & Gard Ltd, Bristol, England
Printed in Great Britain by Clays Ltd, St Ives plc

British Library Cataloguing in Publication Data
Developing communication and counselling skills in medicine.
   1. Medicine. Personnel. Communication with patients
   I. Corney, Roslyn H. (Roslyn Heather) *1948–*
   610.696

Library of Congress Cataloging in Publication Data
Developing communication and counselling skills in medicine / edited
   by Roslyn Corney.
   p.   cm.
   Includes bibliographical references and index.
   1. Physician and patient. 2. Communication in medicine.
   I. Corney, Roslyn H.
   [DNLM: 1. Communication. 2. Counseling—methods. 3. Physician
   –Patient Relations.   W 62 D489]
   R727.3.D47   1991
   610.69'6—dc20
   DNLM/DLC
   for Library of Congress
                                91-18610
                                CIP

ISBN 0-415-04235-6
    0-415-04236-4 (pbk)

To Rex, Rebecca and James

Contents

Contributors

Russell Blacker is a Consultant Psychiatrist at the Royal Cornwall Hospital in Truro. He has a substantial commitment to training GPs and to liaison psychiatry and is involved in specialized clinics including a combined pain and chronic fatigue clinic. Current research includes a study on the psychological consequences of termination of pregnancy, the neuropsychiatric basis of chronic fatigue, deliberate self-harm and antidepressant therapies. He trained at Guys and subsequently at St Bartholomew's Hospital where he completed an MD thesis on Depression in General Practice.

James Calnan was Professor of Plastic and Reconstructive Surgery at the Royal Postgraduate Medical School and Hammersmith Hospital where he worked from 1960 until retirement in 1981 (now Emeritus). He has written extensively on medical research and practical plastic surgery, and has published nine books. At one time he had an extensive medico-legal practice and has acted as adviser to various TV programmes.

Anthony Clare is Medical Director of St Patrick's and Clinical Professor of Psychiatry at Trinity College, Dublin, having been formerly Professor of Psychological Medicine at St Bartholomew's Hospital in London. He has written extensively on relationships between psychiatry and medicine.

Jeremy Coid is a Consultant in Forensic Psychiatry to the North East Thames Regional Health Authority and Senior Lecturer in Forensic Psychiatry to the Medical College of St Bartholomew's Hospital, University of London. He is in charge of a Regional Secure Unit for mentally abnormal offenders in the East End of London. He has carried out research into violent prisoners and patients and has worked in a range of previous settings including prisons and maximum security hospitals.

Roslyn Corney is a Senior Lecturer working in the Department of Psychological Medicine at St Bartholomew's Hospital, in the Department of Psychiatry at the Institute of Psychiatry and in the Centre for Health Service Studies at the University of Kent in Canterbury. A psychologist by training, she has conducted a number of clinical trials of counselling for psychiatric and psychosomatic illness and has conducted a study of the psychological and social adjustment of women after major gynaecological surgery. She is particularly interested in developing the skills of both primary and secondary care practitioners in the identification and management of psychosocial disorders and emotional distress.

Linda Gask is a Senior Research Fellow and Honorary Consultant Psychiatrist in the Departments of Psychiatry and General Practice at the University of Sheffield. She is also a Project Manager for Research and Development for Psychiatry, an organization funded by one of the Sainsbury Family Trusts. Her main interest is in developing training packages for primary care in the fields of communication skills and detection and management of psychosocial problems.

Roger Higgs is a General Practitioner in inner city London and Professor in the Department of General Practice and Primary Care at King's College Hospital Medical School. He has a particular interest in health care ethics, psychosocial issues in primary care and in the development and assessment of innovations in care in the community. He thinks that most professionals in training in health care get a raw deal and would like to see that improved.

Nira Kfir received her Doctorate at the Sorbonne. Her contributions to the field of Psychology have been in the development of her Model of Crisis Intervention and her personality priorities therapy called Impasse/Priority Therapy. Together with Maurice Slevin she has developed her Model into seminars for work with cancer patients. She lectures extensively in England, Europe and the USA. Her book *Crisis Intervention Verbatim* was published by Hemisphere, 1988.

Janice Kohler is a Senior Lecturer in Paediatric Oncology in Southampton. She obtained a medical degree from Bristol University in 1975. After three years in general paediatrics in Wessex she went to Great Ormond Street Hospital for specialist training in paediatric oncology. In Southampton she is involved in teaching and research as well as clinic oncology, and has a husband, two energetic sons and a dog to distract her at home.

Peter Maguire is a Senior Lecturer in Psychiatry in the University Department of Psychiatry at Withington Hospital, South Manchester. He is an honorary Consultant Psychiatrist and also Director of the Cancer Research Campaign Psychological Medicine Group at Stanley House, Christie Hospital, South Manchester. He is particularly interested in developing methods to help patients and relatives cope with cancer and cancer treatment. He is also involved in developing and evaluating methods of training health professionals in basic interviewing, assessment and counselling skills.

Robert Newell is a lecturer in Nursing at Hull University. He has worked in behaviour therapy for the past eight years, most recently as a trainer of nurse behaviour therapists. His chief area of clinical research is in behavioural medicine and he is currently involved in teaching undergraduate nurses, using a cognitive behavioural approach.

Maurice Slevin is a Consultant Physician and Medical Oncologist at both St Bartholomew's Hospital and the Homerton Hospital, London. He is also Chairman of BACUP (British Association of Cancer United Patients).

Averil Stedeford was Consultant in Psychological Medicine at Sir Michael Sobell House, a hospice in Oxford, where she worked for twelve years. Two years ago she left to concentrate on psychotherapy in private practice and she now has an honorary consultant post at the Psychotherapy Department of the Warneford Hospital. She is interested in writing and teaching about terminal care and bereavement and in linking knowledge and practice in this area with psychoanalysis. Her writing includes papers and a book, and most recently a volume of poetry, some of which she uses in teaching.

Jenifer Wilson-Barnett has been Professor and Head of the Department of Nursing Studies at Kings College, London, since 1986. She started her career at St George's Hospital as a student and later staff nurse. She then spent the next decade between academic studies and professional posts. Her research work has involved evaluating psychological interventions for those with physical illness.

Preface

This book has been written for medical students and young doctors engaged in clinical work with patients. The focus of the book is on developing communication skills with patients and will therefore be helpful to nurses and other health professionals whose work involves talking with patients and conducting interviews.

The need to train health professionals in communication skills is now being recognized. Studies of patients' views suggest that many patients are dissatisfied with the interactions with doctors and this is a common cause for patients' complaints. Medical educators are increasingly including skills training in their curriculum and assessments of interview techniques are being made. Research studies indicate that good communication skills can be learnt by students and that with rehearsal and practice they can become an everyday part of interacting with patients.

The book is divided into three parts. The first part deals with more general issues and ideas and the second concentrates on more specific and often difficult situations which health professionals encounter regularly. A number of the chapters in this second section offer detailed guidelines on how to develop specific communication skills and techniques using case examples. The third section focuses on the needs of the clinician and the importance of looking after oneself as well as briefly outlining some of the important agencies and voluntary groups working in this area.

In the text the patient and the doctor are sometimes referred to as 'he' and sometimes 'she'. This is merely a convenience of style as it is considered less cumbersome than always using the term 'they' or 'he/she'.

Thanks are due to colleagues in the Department of Psychological Medicine at St Bartholomew's Hospital, London, and the Section of Epidemiology and General Practice, Institute of Psychiatry. I would also like to thank Julie Smith for her conscientious typing of the manuscript.

Part I

Basic issues and skills

Chapter 1

The need for better communication and emotional support

Roslyn Corney

In the twentieth century, health care has changed dramatically with the rapid growth in knowledge in the medical sciences as well as the development of sophisticated diagnostic and treatment facilities. There has also been a change in priorities in health care. Infectious diseases have been reduced to be replaced by an increase in chronic and degenerative problems. This has led to an increase in long-term treatments with the emphasis on control rather than cure. These treatments need active participation and involvement from the patient. As they are long-term, attention also needs to be paid to social and psychological factors as well as physical problems.

It is important that the training of medical and other health workers does not become too focused on the technological and biomedical dimensions of health care to the exclusion of a more holistic view of the patient. One major task of health care is to provide reassurance and comfort for those in distress about their illness. There is also a need to provide the patient with an explanation for illness as well as instructions as to how best to deal with it. Giving such information and support may be one of the most important tasks performed by the doctor.

Although a number of studies have amply demonstrated the importance of good communication skills, it has only been relatively recently that attention has been paid to developing interviewing and communication skills in medical education. It is perhaps assumed that these skills will come with practice and by observing the interactions of experienced doctors. Yet dissatisfaction with medical communication is one of the most common of patients' complaints. It is also a major factor why some patients choose other forms of help and treatment, such as alternative medicine, with its focus on actively involving the patient in treatment and encouraging them to talk freely about their problems.

This chapter focuses on the need for better communication, information and emotional support for patients. These skills are needed:

1   in the process of diagnosis and treatment. This includes the doctor ascertaining the patient's concerns, worries and theories about the illness and responding appropriately.
2   to give information to the patient regarding their illness, its treatment and any side effects and making sure that these have been understood and remembered.
3   to give emotional support and care to patients and their families, recognizing their feelings, fears, distress and anxiety.

DIAGNOSIS AND TREATMENT

When individuals become ill, their concerns, preoccupations and worries change dramatically, focusing around the illness and the effect it may have on their daily activities, their work and their family life. It is important that the doctor is aware of the need to attend to psychological factors and is alerted to the worries and distress of his patient. A failure to discuss these problems means that the doctor and patient are concerned with different priorities and that good communication is unlikely.

While most medical encounters are initiated by patients, the purpose of the meeting may be very different for the patient than for the doctor. For example, the purpose from the patients' point of view may be to seek relief from pain or discomfort, to obtain a sickness certificate, or to receive reassurance about their health. The doctor, on the other hand, may see the purpose of the interview is to reach an accurate diagnosis or prescribe appropriate treatment. The doctor may regard the interview purely as a process in which information is extracted and therefore interpersonal issues are unimportant. He may not consider the patient's need for reassurance, for example. However, without this assurance, the patient may consult again with exactly the same anxieties.

Elicit the patient's theories

Another important facet of interviewing is to elicit the patient's own theories about his illness or symptoms. Patients bring to the consultation their own ideas which may be very different to the doctor's. It is important that the doctor discovers these theories and either confirms them or rules them out by discussing them with the patient. Failure to discuss these theories may leave the patient confused, not knowing what to believe. This conflict in the patient will affect the patient's compliance with treatment and his satisfaction with the consultation.

Doctor- or patient-centred

The first problem presented by patients may not be their major problem and a sensitive doctor can seek out the 'real' problem by attending to a variety of verbal and non-verbal cues presented by the patient.

In one study over 2,000 general practice consultations were tape-recorded. The authors classified three-quarters of the interviews as doctor-centred. In these the doctor concentrated on questions about the first complaint presented by the patient. They quickly achieved an organic diagnosis and usually gave a prescription. They often ignored verbal or non-verbal leads about other problems presented. The remaining quarter of the doctors were more patient-centred. With these, the doctor took a less controlling role enabling the patient to give an account of symptoms, worries and fears. Patient-centred doctors were more apt to ask 'open' questions which did not restrict the answers given by patients. Open questions give the patient the option of introducing new theories or facts rather than just confirming the hypotheses generated by the doctor. 'Closed' questions were used more often by the doctor-centred doctors; these are questions answered by either a 'yes' or 'no'.

The study found that the doctors tended to have consistent interviewing styles and used a set of interview behaviours whatever problem was presented to them. It has been suggested that doctors develop their interviewing style early on in their careers, possibly adopting that of their tutors, and that subsequent experience does not alter their behaviour.

The Los Angeles studies

A number of studies of doctor–patient interaction were conducted at the Childrens' Hospital in Los Angeles in the late 1960s and the 1970s. In these studies, tape-recordings were made of 800 successive consultations between doctors and mothers who had brought their children to a clinic. The clinic was specifically for acute disorders and consultations tended to be short. The doctors studied were full-time members of staff, they were young and well-trained paediatricians. Mothers were interviewed immediately after the consultation concerning their expectations and their degree of satisfaction.

Many of the mothers experienced difficulties in getting the doctors to understand their real concerns and worries. Most mothers were subjected to a number of questions which often did not seem to them to be related to the child's symptoms. While the doctor may have had a clear idea of the hypotheses which he was testing, he had not conveyed this adequately to the mother which had left her confused and often dissatisfied. One quarter of the mothers said that they had not mentioned their greatest concern to the doctor, because the opportunity hadn't occurred or because he hadn't asked them to. The doctor was thus attempting to decide on his diagnosis along lines which he understood, while the mother was so involved in her own problems and concerns that she could not adequately focus on what she was being asked and told to do.

These studies indicate the need for openness on the part of the doctor and to show an interest in the patient's concerns and their viewpoints regarding treatment. The doctor, after eliciting this information from the patient, has to give clear information to the patient about his illness and treatment. He also has to make sure that this is given in a form that is both understood by the patient and easily remembered.

THE NEED FOR INFORMATION

Many studies have indicated that patients are left confused after they have seen their doctor as the doctor failed to give clear diagnostic and prognostic statements. The patient's confusion may be due to their own anxiety, distress or preoccupations. These may affect the patient's ability to concentrate on what has been said. In addition, the confusion may be due to the doctor being unclear in some way. This can be due to a number of reasons, for example, the doctor may:

1   be unclear or unsure about the diagnosis or the prognosis.
2   be rushed and have little time to explain the situation fully.
3   find it difficult to break 'bad news' or unsavoury information and therefore cope by avoiding the issue.
4   not realize the importance of giving information in this case.
5   withhold information as he feels it best that the patient does not know what is wrong as this will only disturb and distress him.
6   be fearful of becoming emotionally involved, so he avoids any communicative contact that may become emotional.

Ley (1988) in his review of the literature suggests that there is no evidence of increased anxiety or depression when patients are told of their diagnosis. Even studies of cancer patients suggest that the majority of patients would prefer to be informed although there is still some debate whether all patients should be told. Surveys indicate that most patients wish to know as much as possible about their illness, its causes, treatments and outcome.

Reviews of studies on a range of surgical patients show generally positive results of giving adequate information and preparation before surgery. Preparation has been shown to affect post-operative pain and symptoms, time taken to recover as well as anxiety levels.

EMOTIONAL SUPPORT AND CARE

Distress and anxiety

The different reactions that patients have to illness is discussed in the next chapter. Whatever they may be, it is important that the doctor responds to them, acknowledges them and takes them into account when he communicates with the patient.

The most common reactions of patients to illness are distress and anxiety. Overall estimates suggest that between 30 and 60 per cent of general hospital patients suffer significant levels of psychological distress at the time of hospitalization and during the first year afterwards. In addition, general practice studies suggest that between 10 and 30 per cent of all their consultations are for psychosocial reasons.

Distress is also common among relatives which in turn affects the patient. In a study on patients suffering from coronary heart disease, 80 per cent of patients and half of their spouses revealed mild or moderate distress while in hospital and approximately half of the patients and spouses still felt distressed two months later.

It is important to respond to this distress and anxiety by acknowledgement and support. This is not only for humanitarian reasons but because it has been found that the presence of psychological distress has a negative effect on recovery from illness. In a large scale survey, Querido studied 1,630 patients admitted to a hospital in Amsterdam. Six months after discharge, 70 per cent of patients who were classified as distressed whilst in hospital were in an unsatisfactory condition medically in comparison with only 30 per cent of those classified as non-distressed. While 1,128 of the 1,630 patients had been given a favourable medical prognosis, only 660 had lived up to this expectation. The majority of those who failed to improve had been classified as distressed while in hospital.

Other studies have indicated that psychological responses affect survival. Greer and colleagues found that women's attitudes and reactions to breast cancer affected their survival rate. Women whose reactions to cancer were either a fighting spirit or denial survived better than those who were distressed, felt hopeless, or helpless. Of the women who subsequently died, 88 per cent reacted with stoic acceptance or helplessness/hopelessness whereas only 46 per cent of the women who remained alive and well had demonstrated these reactions.

Reducing distress and anxiety

Distress and anxiety can be reduced in a number of ways. It is often uncertainty which is the most difficult to bear and distress can be reduced by providing information about the illness and treatment. Studies have also indicated that emotional distress can be reduced by actively involving the patient in treatment and decisions regarding treatment. The patient regards himself as being actively involved in treating or fighting the illness rather than feeling passive and helpless.

It is also important, however, not only to give information but to acknowledge the distress felt by the patient and to offer support, sympathy and reassurance. In the Los Angeles studies, statements of feeling worried or tense accounted for 10 per cent of the parents' utterances. Nevertheless, doctors rarely responded with reassurance. The most common complaint from dissatisfied mothers was the doctor's lack of sympathy. The tape recordings confirm that the doctors' conversations with the parent were rarely friendly (less than 6 per cent) although they were generally more friendly and warm towards the child. The doctors were perhaps aware that friendliness was important to elicit cooperation from the child but did not rate this as important with the parent. For most of the consultations the doctors paid no attention to the mothers' feelings and confined their conversation to a discussion about their children's condition. These doctors perceived their responsibility was to identify and treat the disease, rather than treat the parent or their child.

The Los Angeles studies also found that one of the strongest determinants of compliance with treatment was satisfaction with the consultation. Mothers were visited at home within fourteen days of the consultation with the paediatrician to see if they had complied with the advice they had been given. They found that patients who considered that the interview was satisfactory were three times as likely to have complied than those who regarded the consultation unsatisfactory. While parents rarely disagreed with the doctor during the consultation, once home they treated their children as they thought best rather than according to the advice given.

WHY DOCTORS ARE SOMETIMES POOR AT COMMUNICATION

Despite the evidence of the importance of good information, communication and emotional support, doctors have been criticized for their neglect of this area. This could be partly due to the lack of communication skills training on the medical curriculum. However, it has often been said that the only way that doctors can bear the burden of clinical responsibility and remain objective while making decisions is by distancing themselves from any of the distressing consequences. In addition, caring and compassion by doctors is sometimes actively discouraged; in some cases, doctors have been trained to remain detached.

However, for the many reasons listed earlier, it is important that doctors are not cut off from the emotional needs of the patients. Training will help the process of enabling the doctor to cope but doctors should perhaps consider the need for support for themselves. Workers in other caring professions, such as counselling and social work, have supervision sessions built into their work. In these meetings, they are given support and help to disentangle their own feelings, avoidances, prejudices and emotional responses.

Training in communication skills

Students cannot easily learn good interviewing techniques by unsupervised practice. In addition, they may pick up bad habits and poor interviewing styles from senior staff. Often students are given forms for history-taking thus indicating that obtaining factual information from the patient is all that is necessary. In addition, students will find it difficult to talk about personal and emotional issues to patients because they are unsure about how to approach the subject or because they are frightened about what might happen if they do.

One study found that students did not always learn better communication skills by experience. He found that students became less interested in their patients as people over time. Senior students were less likely than junior students to question patients on psychological or social dimensions. Students therefore became more doctor-centred as they progressed through medical school.

However, the process is not irreversible. Thompson and Anderson (1982) found that after a tutorial, students were significantly better at introducing themselves, preparing the patient for the interview, asking clear open simple questions, giving explanations and terminating the interview appropriately. They found patients preferred students who were easy to talk to and confide in, sympathetic and warm. They also preferred students who avoided repetition, who gave appropriate encouragement, who were aware of verbal leads and who were self-assured and precise.

This study and others suggest that communication skills can be learnt. However, awareness of the need to develop these skills must come first. After this, tutorials, discussion of techniques and actual interviews, together with the use of video, audio and direct observation of the student's performance can all have an enabling role.

SUGGESTED FURTHER READING

Ley, P. (1988) *Communicating with Patients*, London: Croom Helm.

Nichols, K.A. (1984) *Psychological Care in Physical Illness*, London: Croom Helm.

Rutter, D.R. and Maguire, G. (1976) 'History taking for medical students: II. Evaluation of a training programme', *Lancet* 1: 558–60.

Thompson, J.A. and Anderson, J.L. (1982) 'Patient preferences and the bedside manner', *Medical Education* 16: 17–21.

Tuckett, D.A., Boulton, M., Olson, C. and Williams, A. (1986) *Meetings Between Experts: an approach to sharing ideas in medical consultations*, London: Tavistock Publications.

Chapter 2

Emotional responses in patients and doctors

Roslyn Corney

This chapter will introduce the sorts of feelings aroused in patients by becoming ill and by being in hospital. These include fear, shock, denial, depression, shame, guilt or anger. It will also briefly discuss the common feelings felt by health care professionals involved, their fears, worries and distress which often stop them adopting a more caring and communicative attitude.

Many of these emotions felt by patients and the professionals involved will be discussed in more detail in later chapters including guidance on how best to respond.

EMOTIONAL REACTIONS TO ILLNESS AND WAYS OF COPING

A number of factors, such as personality and age will affect how an individual responds to becoming ill. These responses are characteristic of that individual's usual response to stress and are not specific to any particular illness or disease. Some people will attempt to ignore the signs and symptoms of illness, hoping that they will disappear of their own accord. Others trivialize the magnitude of the symptoms while others become withdrawn and depressed. Certain patients may welcome the symptoms of illness as it is one way of avoiding certain situations or responsibilities.

In addition, the subject's previous experience of illness should also be taken into account. For example, previous experience of similar problems can reduce anxiety because there is less uncertainty. On the other hand if the patient has seen similar symptoms in a close friend or relative who has had a more serious illness, then groundless fears may occur.

The patient's psychological state at the time of the illness also plays a major part in determining how severe the illness is perceived to be. Anxiety can reduce pain tolerance and studies have suggested that anxiety rather than symptom frequency or severity is a critical factor in determining whether an individual seeks medical attention. Sometimes a particular part of the body can have a particular significance for the patient. Mastectomy may be particularly disturbing for many women, especially those who rate physical attractiveness highly or those involved in fragile relationships. In general, disabling disorders are often perceived as more threatening by men whereas women react more strongly to disfiguring diseases.

Reactions of the family and friends also play a role. Recovery from illness tends to be quicker in those who have good social support or who are involved in loving relationships. However, there are often major problems experienced by families in caring for a member, particularly with a chronic illness. It is important for the family to be adequately involved and prepared for dealing with the long-term demands.

ANXIETY

Illness produces a number of fears in patients, including the fear of pain, disability and death. Anxieties are often at their most intense when there is uncertainty regarding a diagnosis or illness. Many patients find the period of time before diagnosis to be the most stressful period. Once they know what is wrong with them, they can start to accept this and plan accordingly.

Patients may also have unrealistic fears. Certain individuals are phobic about certain illnesses or specific forms of treatment. Cancerphobia is common. It is therefore important that the doctor finds out the patient's particular worries, so that appropriate reassurance may be given.

Usually talking about such concerns to a sympathetic and supportive person will help reduce these feelings. Many individuals, however, find it difficult to talk about their fears or anxieties. Men, in particular, are taught from childhood not to show their emotions. It may be helpful to suggest that fear or anxiety are common responses to being ill or being in hospital thus 'allowing' the patient to talk about them.

The anxious patient may be difficult to interview until the anxiety itself has been discussed. Anxieties are also likely to be reduced when patients receive full and complete explanations to their questions.

DENIAL

It is not uncommon for patients to show initial denial as a way of coping. This may be protective allowing the patient to get through the early stages of the illness after diagnosis. However, some patients continue with this denial, they cope by either refusing to believe that they are ill or by trivializing the illness.

These patients may misinform and mislead the doctor, as they will consistently minimize symptoms or sometimes deny they exist. If patients dismiss all symptoms as minor, the doctor should consider the possibility of denial and try to interview a reliable relative or informant.

There is some evidence that denial can be an adaptive mechanism. Greer's work on reactions to breast cancer and survival and studies on coronary care units suggest that denial can be protective. However denial can become dangerous when individuals ignore the early signs of a serious disease such as cancer and delay seeking medical help.

Methods of dealing with denial are included in Chapter 6, 'Managing difficult communication tasks'.

DEPRESSION

One of the commonest reported responses to illness is that of depression. This can be so intense that patients become weepy, withdraw and even contemplate suicide. Depressed people have feelings of guilt, worthlessness, and hopelessness. This may be manifested in the patient's manner, appearance, tone of voice, posture and speech.

Depression is most prevalent after the initial stages of an illness when the individual is coming to terms with the full implications of being ill. It may be associated with a sense of loss of physical or social functioning. Depression may also arise from feelings of guilt, patients perceiving their illness as a punishment for past behaviour. Sometimes guilty patients become passive believing that their punishment is justified. These patients may show little motivation towards treatment and recovery and can be difficult to treat.

Some people respond to illness by a feeling of hopelessness and helplessness. They can become passive and withdrawn. These patients often have a poor physical prognosis failing to fight back against the illness or to be seriously committed to participation in treatment.

It is often helpful to draw attention to the fact that the patient 'looks very upset or sad'. This will give the patient the opportunity to talk about his feelings. As with anxiety, this may be necessary before discussion of the illness proceeds. With severe depression, psychiatric help may be necessary.

Crying

Most doctors find it uncomfortable when a patient cries during the interview. The release of emotion, however, may be of considerable help both to patient and interviewer. Weeping often brings some relief to the patient making it possible for the patient to talk afterwards. It may also help develop the relationship between patient and doctor.

A common mistake in these situations is for the clinician to interrupt the crying with a remark such as 'you will soon feel better' or 'time heals'; this is often due to the clinician's discomfort and feelings of embarrassment. Instead, it is better to wait until the patient has stopped crying and then respond sympathetically. It can be helpful at this time to point out how unhappy they must feel rather than to ignore the feelings. Being given the opportunity to cry followed by a supportive and sympathetic response can be very helpful to the patient.

ANGER

There are many things that provoke anger in a patient. The patient will be angry at being ill and by all the distress and problems this causes himself and his family. In addition, anger can be an appropriate response to being ill or being a patient in hospital. Waiting to be seen and the uncaring attitudes of certain staff are common occurrences. In addition, patients who are anxious may respond with anger more readily than they would in more normal circumstances.

Dealing with a patient's anger is dealt with in Chapter 6, 'Managing difficult communication tasks'. However, as with depression or anxiety, it is usually helpful to draw attention to the patient's emotions by a sympathetic remark rather than by avoidance.

ACTIVE COPING

Some patients cope with their anxiety by finding out as much as possible about the nature of their illness and its treatment. Information is particularly important for these patients and active involvement and participation in treatment should be encouraged as long as it is not carried to extremes. For example, patients may discover their own ways of dealing with the limitations imposed by the illness. This will make these individuals feel that they are doing something constructive rather than being passive. These individuals often wish to be in control and be prepared for future events. They may benefit from being involved in patient groups and can be of great help to others in the same situation.

THE STRESS OF BEING IN HOSPITAL

In addition to the stress of becoming ill, being admitted to hospital is often regarded by patients as being one of the most stressful events of their life. Admission to hospital removes the individual from his family, relatives and friends and places him in an unfamiliar environment which is often seen by patients as clinical, impersonal and cold. Patients find themselves restricted and may have to spend a considerable amount of time confined to bed. In hospital, most privacy and independence will be lost. Eating and sleeping will be carried out in the presence of strangers. In addition, the patient has little control over the daily routine, which is very likely to be different from home, and the patient has to learn to adjust.

Many people fear going into hospital. This fear may be greater than their fear of the illness. Some of this anxiety is related to uncertainty about treatment. Many medical procedures give rise to considerable discomfort and anxiety. Strange people observe, move and treat various parts of their bodies. While medical staff may regard procedures or operations as routine, they may cause a considerable amount of anxiety to the patient.

Some of the more common feelings associated with anxiety are those of helplessness or fears of dependency. These are normal in hospital situations. The surgical patient knows that for a period of time before, during and after the operation, he will be totally helpless. For most individuals being dependent for a short period of time does not pose difficulties. However, for some individuals the need to be independent and active is very strong and to be cared for is quite intolerable.

Efforts should be made to reduce the patient's sense of helplessness by allowing him to be as active as the situation permits and to be involved in as many decisions as possible. Allowing the patient some control over his daily activities or choice over his situation will help.

THE DOCTOR'S EMOTIONAL RESPONSE TO SPECIFIC PATIENTS

Doctors will respond differently according to the characteristics of their patients. These feelings are normal and natural but it is important to be aware of them. It is possible to make mistakes when these feelings are acted upon but are not recognized.

Doctors' attitudes towards certain patients can reflect previously learned attitudes. For example a doctor may feel awkward when interviewing patients who are similar in some way to his own parents. He may find it difficult to ask relevant personal questions. Alternatively, a doctor may find he is strongly attracted to a patient. These interactions between doctor and patient may have strong emotional undercurrents which can affect the doctor's judgement.

These subjective feelings are often not discussed with others. However, subjective reactions occurring must be acknowledged so that they do not interfere with patient care. For instance, one may be feeling angry, depressed or irritable before seeing a patient but it is important not to let these feelings be transferred into the consultation or projected on to the patient.

Doctors may feel uneasy about provoking angry, distressing or embarrassing scenes and avoid situations where this might happen. For this reason, they may find it difficult to mention specific topics which they think patients might not want to divulge. This could include topics such as suicidal thoughts, termination of pregnancy, or homosexuality.

Other doctors find it difficult to cope with emotional distress and may avoid telling patients bad news or leave the situation as soon as possible afterwards, failing to give adequate support to the patient. A further kind of emotional scene that a doctor may seek to avoid is any display of discord, either involving himself or occurring between other people such as the patient and their spouse.

Topics which the doctor finds most difficult to discuss are often those in which he is experiencing some difficulty himself. If the difficulty in his patient's life is similar to some unresolved problem within himself, the doctor will have problems discussing the situation calmly and objectively. The doctor may be unhappily married or feel guilty about an extra-marital affair. The doctor may respond by avoiding any discussions on the topic with the patient or by denying its importance. Thus unresolved difficulties and conflicts can affect the doctor's ability to communicate sensitively.

Experiencing difficulties and problems, however, may not always have negative effects. If these conflicts are resolved in some way, the doctor's own experiences can sometimes provide him with greater insight into the problems of his patient and increase his sensitivity.

Common reactions

Anxiety is common in doctors as well as patients. It is not always easy not to worry about whether one has made the right decisions regarding diagnosis or treatment. It is often difficult to admit to fears or feelings of inadequacy. Students are usually trained to exhibit the opposite behaviour, always being in control, self-confident, without any doubts.

As with patients, there are some doctors whose way of dealing with emotional and strong feelings is to deny them, thus protecting themselves. The doctor may consider that his own feelings are best ignored or restrained. However, this in turn may lead the doctor to ignore the feelings of his patients and to refuse to enter into discussions about these emotions.

Despair is another common reaction. The more dedicated a doctor is to curing patients, the more difficult he may find having to be involved with patients with terminal illness. Many doctors cope with these feelings of despair and helplessness by avoiding the patient or avoiding emotional issues. Another reaction is overtreatment. This can raise the hopes of patients and families as well as increase the medical interventions that they have to endure. Alternatively, the doctor may react by rejection, referring the patient elsewhere. All of these reactions are usually detrimental to the patient.

Many of these themes will be discussed in greater length in later chapters; the doctor's own feelings and responses are explored in Chapter 14, 'Looking after yourself'.

SUGGESTED FURTHER READING

Enelow, A.J. and Swisher, S.N. (1986) *Interviewing and Patient Care*, 3rd edn, Oxford: Oxford University Press.

Greer, S., Morris, T. and Pettingale, K.W. (1979) 'Psychological response to breast cancer: effect on outcome', *Lancet* 1: 785–7.

Chapter 3

Developing communication and interviewing skills

Anthony Clare

INTRODUCTION

Elsewhere in this book the need for better communication in medicine is described – to facilitate better diagnosis and treatment, to provide comprehensive information for patients and relatives, to manage difficult situations – the underlying premise being that today's clinician, whatever his speciality and wherever he practises, requires to be a competent interviewer and a skilful communicator. This chapter examines how such abilities and skills can be developed. Underpinning the process is the relationship between the doctor and the patient, its nature and the expectations each brings to bear upon it. There are, of course, interview techniques and styles which can turn a prosaic interview into a competent one but just how the two participants relate often holds the key to success.

THE DOCTOR–PATIENT RELATIONSHIP

There are a number of important features of the relationship between doctor and patient including the patient's trust and confidence in the physician and the autonomy of the patient. Illnesses that lead people to seek help are more often than not accompanied by anxiety, feelings of helplessness and disruption in the patient's normal relationships with those around him. Illness can evoke fears of financial troubles or occupational difficulties; sometimes illness is provoked by such or similar stresses. The patient can come to the doctor bearing not merely the symptoms of a particular illness but considerable worry about possible causes and effects. Mixed up with such worries is hope that something can be done and that not merely will health be restored but so too will the patient's ability to cope and control his life once more.

With certain symptoms there may be particular worries – about the possibility of serious illness, of being incapacitated, of having to experience great pain or undergo frightening tests. Some symptoms can be embarrassing and the patient may find that having buoyed himself up to unburden himself he actually cannot give a full account of what ails him without a good deal of encouragement and understanding on the part of the doctor.

Such understandable anxiety actually provides the doctor with a valuable opportunity to demonstrate his professional skills and his clinical understanding at the very outset. Putting patients at their ease and letting them say what worries them is a most potent way of winning patients' confidence. The ability of the doctor to be aware of and cue into the patient's anxiety suggests to the patient that he is in the hands of a true professional. Merely for the doctor to acknowledge the possibility of anxiety on the part of the patient can help. Conversely, any suggestion of lack of time, of impatience, of a lack of sympathy or sensitivity to how the patient is feeling at the outset of the interview can undermine the subsequent relationship in a grievous way.

Everyday clinical reality, of course, means that doctors do find themselves pressed for time, irritated by what seem excessive demands and frustrated by patients who are as ready to ignore advice as they are to seek it. In such circumstances, it may be tempting to be brusque, impatient and matter-of-fact. For the sake of the ultimate outcome of the interview such temptation is usually best avoided.

The nature of the doctor–patient relationship varies. Three types have been described by Szasz and Hollender: activity–passivity, guidance–cooperation and mutual participation. The degree of participation and the feeling of autonomy on the part of the patient are the two main variables in these three types of relationship.

In the *activity–passivity* type of relationship, the doctor exploits all the authority and control inherent in his status while the patient experiences and wields no autonomy. The patient does not actively participate in treatment but accepts what is decided. Such an arrangement is appropriate in emergency situations in which rapid decisions of a professional kind have to be made and implemented but it is highly inappropriate when diagnostic interviewing, data gathering and treatment are involved. The activity–passivity model of interviewing involves the doctor asking all the questions and the patient answering them in a model that closely resembles a legal cross-examination in a courtroom – it is an approach which may be all very well when a doctor is struggling to establish a set of facts such as the basic demographic data relating to a patient – but it is cold and counter-productive when the doctor is trying to establish how the patient is feeling.

In the *guidance–cooperation* type of doctor–patient relationship the doctor still wields considerable authority but the patient experiences a greater degree of personal autonomy and is able to participate somewhat more actively. This approach, while more effective in putting the patient at ease, still restricts the agenda of the discussion to what the doctor wants. The patient's desire to please the doctor may still lead to a partial account of problems. For example, the doctor may focus on a particular set of symptoms and indicate to the patient that he has all the time in the world to discuss these. However, while the patient may feel that there is another symptom altogether which worries him more or which he feels is for some other reason more important he none the less keeps it to himself because it does not appear to figure on the doctor's agenda for discussion. The patient is indeed required to collaborate and actively participate in this relationship model but the terms of the relationship are still laid down by the doctor.

The *mutual participation* relationship is usually the most desirable for the interview leading towards a diagnosis, for the management of chronic and disabling illnesses and for the resolution of anxiety and tension related to the interview itself. In this model, doctor and patient are expected to behave as active participants and to exercise personal responsibility and the patient is encouraged to feel some responsibility for the successful completion of the interview. The doctor has to acknowledge the reality of his professional status and authority if only to make explicit to the patient that they are of very much less importance in the interview setting given the nature of the aims of the interview and its desired outcome. For example, the patient can readily grasp the importance of his role if he is reminded at intervals that without his collaboration or his detailed account of how he feels or his personal perspective concerning his illness or treatment or social circumstances the doctor's professional status and skills are relatively impaired. Of course it is true that some degree of dependence on the doctor is inevitable and is often useful, for example in acute, potentially frightening diseases where it can be used to help the doctor reassure and relieve the patient. But it can also be a nuisance, encouraging patients to regard the doctor, medical technology and all sorts of other external factors as the road to cure and their own role in the healing process as negligible or even non-existent. Worse, undue dependence can lead to a situation in which the patient believes that without regular access to the doctor he cannot survive – and such a relationship by virtue of such dependence is in the final analysis anti-therapeutic.

Depending on the purpose of the interview, the circumstances in which it is carried out and factors relating to the patient's problems, these three relationships will be variously exploited. It is one of the tasks of a physician to be able to establish a doctor–patient relationship or modify an existing one so that its characteristics are appropriate for the patient to resolve conflicts and difficulties within it.

In what way do expectations affect the doctor–patient relationship? In general, patients expect doctors to be interested, compassionate, reassuring, sensitive and skilful. If patients are particularly distressed they are exceptionally vulnerable and their expectations of care and compassion all the more intense. There is the expectation too that the culmination of the interview will be some feeling of relief as well as the absence of discomfort or pain. Doctors should attend to such expectations and where it is feasible attempt to fulfil them. Where the doctor identifies unrealistic expectations (of, for example, a dramatic cure when what is being presented is a chronic, intractable problem) he should acknowledge the gap and encourage the patient to examine the discrepancy between ideal and reality. Open and frank discussions about treatment and prognosis are usually helpful but in most instances can only be undertaken with confidence and safety if some degree of trust and confidence between doctor and patient has already been established.

There can be negative expectations of the doctor too. Patients who have seen many doctors, who have undergone many treatments, who have failed to respond to earlier interventions may well begin a new consultation with distinctly negative expectations. Patients can project on to the authority figure of the doctor resentments and hostility resulting from experiences of authority figures in the patient's own life. Obvious examples include patients who are themselves the offspring of parents working the the 'caring' profession – if such patients have reason to be somewhat ambivalent or indeed downright cynical about their parents' caring for them they may take such ambivalence and hostility and wrap it around any representative figure of the caring professions they encounter during their sick-role state.

Doctors who do not attend to such a possibility are often puzzled by the intensity of the negative emotions directed at them at the outset of an interview. It is in this sense that it is true to say that every doctor at the outset of a clinical interview is on trial – patients are keen to establish which kind of doctor he is, the comparison being made in terms of the myriad of fantasies about doctors and equivalent figures which occur in our culture – the doctor as healer, scientist, bureaucrat, experimenter, number-cruncher, businessman, charlatan, healer, God, devil and incompetent.

INTERVIEWING STYLE

An *open-ended interviewing style* is most likely to create the type of clinical relationship desired. It is also the form of interview which is the most effective and efficient way of collecting information about the patient. Doctors tend to seek information in the most direct and economic way possible – a series of specific questions leading to yes/no answers. The doctor usually has a long series of questions which he wishes to ask relating to specific pieces of information. Each piece of information obtained in turn provokes a further series of questions. The interview evolves into an interrogation with the patient becoming more and more passive. Indeed patients who try to communicate personal concerns at first will cease in the later stages of the interview. As a result, important diagnostic information and clues may fail to be elicited.

Open-ended interviewing avoids such a result. More attention is paid to the material which the interviewee wishes to communicate and less to data collection *per se*. There are a number of characteristics of open-ended interviewing (more specific aspects are dealt with in Chapter 5). These include:

1   The interviewer's behaviour should encourage the reduction of tension and the facilitation of communication.
2   The interviewer should attend closely to the nonverbal as well as the verbal behaviour of the interviewee.
3   Information-seeking should be loosely focused and open-ended initially and as the interview proceeds become more tightly focused and directive.

In addition, the interview should be carried out in a private, congenial and comfortable setting if possible where there are few or no interruptions. This is so that free spontaneous behaviour can be encouraged.

BARRIERS TO COMMUNICATION

The major barriers to good communication are status differences (affecting what is termed 'social distance' between the participants), cultural differences and linguistic differences.

Social distance

The interviewing task is made more difficult the wider the social distance between doctor and patient. The patient's trust and cooperation will be influenced by his social class, age, race and culture and the attitudes he brings to the doctor–patient relationship. Likewise, the doctor will carry into the interview attitudes and possibly stereotypes of patients of specific classes, cultures or ethnic groups. It is incumbent on health care professionals, such as doctors, nurses, social workers, psychologists, health visitors, etc., to examine themselves carefully concerning how their attitudes, prejudices and values affect their behaviour. The doctor must also anticipate the patient's own attitudes, suspicions and behaviour. A patient who is afraid of the doctor or who has marked feelings of social inferiority is less likely to ask questions or initiate discussion.

Different cultures

The opportunity for misunderstanding arising out of the fact that doctor and patient come from different cultural backgrounds is substantial. In some cultures, patients are expected to be more passive, doctors more directive. In others, most notably the North American culture, patients can be quite overtly assertive, questioning and spontaneous. Working in a multi-ethnic setting demands that interviewers take account of particular cultural biases. Quite apart from the different emphases placed in different cultures on different symptoms, there can be quite marked variation in such matters as the way emotion is expressed, the degree of stoicism and denial and the expectations concerning the doctor's area of interest. With regard to the last, patients from certain cultures are not affected by the doctor asking intimate questions, e.g. concerning sexuality as a routine part of the general interview. Patients from other cultures, however, may well deduce that since sexual questions are being asked the doctor suspects a sexual problem exists.

Linguistic differences

Quite apart from the problems posed by patients who do not speak the language of the interviewing doctor, the consultation can be seriously compromised by differences in the competence with which doctor and patient communicate in a shared language. In general, doctors are well advised to avoid slang, euphemisms, local phraseology, colloquialisms and abbreviations. Doctors often forget that patients do not have access to medical jargon. Some of the most commonly used terms in medicine – coronary infarction, paralytic ileus, toxic confusional state, dementia – are poorly understood by the general public. Other terms, such as depression, stress, nervous breakdown, schizophrenia, hysterical, have different meanings for the public and professionals. In those circumstances where technical terms have to be used, the doctor should take particular care to explain their meaning and significance.

THE CONSULTATION

In undertaking a clinical interview, there is a variety of tasks the doctor must attend to. These include:

Having a rough plan of the interview   It is useful if the doctor has a rough plan of the interview in his mind, a plan which can be quickly modified in the light of what the patient reveals.

Persuading the patient to talk   This requires that the doctor provides the time and the opportunity for even the most timid or suspicious patient to begin to articulate the problem.

Controlling and guiding the patient with encouragement and appropriate questioning   Any tendency on the part of the patient to garrulousness, over-inclusiveness, obsessional reporting or circumstantiality should be gently curbed.

Recording the salient features of the interview   Occasionally it may be helpful to report verbatim what the patient says but usually a summary is sufficient. However, the doctor needs to avoid seeming to pay more attention to the need to record the patient's problems rather than to attend to them.

Arriving at a diagnosis   Usually the doctor has to come to some conclusion concerning what it is the patient has told him. In so far as there is uncertainty, it may be necessary to indicate this or at least to make clear that further information may be required by way of, for example, physical examination, laboratory tests, third-party interviews, access to other notes, etc.

Summarizing and making decisions on treatment   At the conclusion of the interview, the patient expects a summary of the findings. In most instances, this will require not merely information about what is wrong but what the prognosis is and what treatment is required. Some patients, however, do not want to know about the diagnosis and prognosis while others, in contrast, will want as much information as possible. What the doctor needs to discover is the patient's wishes in this regard, and it may be necessary for the doctor to seek this information on a number of occasions in the interview and not just once.

The discussion should be clear and straightforward. The significance of any findings should be clarified. If there are areas of uncertainty it may be necessary to admit to these. It is important, however, that patients are not overloaded with information and the doctor should be alert to any indication that the patient is not attending or has misunderstood. Many patients consider it impolite or inappropriate to interrupt the doctor for clarification or to reveal that they had not understood. It can be helpful to ask the patient to summarize what they have been told which quickly reveals the extent to which what has been said has been understood.

Eliciting the patient's feelings   Throughout the interview the doctor should be sensitive to how the patient is feeling. When a patient does express feelings the doctor should be quick to provide support; it is unwise to challenge a patient's feelings save in the most extreme circumstances (e.g. when what is said appears to conflict with how the patient appears or behaves). The doctor should resist the temptation to argue with patients about feelings of anger, despair, resentment, rejection, etc., a temptation which can be very pressing if the doctor feels threatened, criticized or attacked by what the patient is saying. Indicating empathy with revealed feelings suggests to the patient that the doctor understands what is going on and such reassurance is important, particularly if the patient has been anticipating rejection or bewilderment. Some patients are reluctant to reveal feelings lest they be ridiculed or dismissed. Indeed one way of encouraging patients to be more forthcoming is explicitly to acknowledge how difficult it can be to reveal feelings of anxiety or self-consciousness. Some of those patients who are most fearful or anxious find it particularly difficult to ask questions and may need help to relax first. Often the less information somebody already has about a condition or treatment the less they ask for.

Some patients are desperate for reassurance and an honest reassurance giving a conservatively phased prediction can decrease anxiety. However, it may not be possible to provide such reassurance after only one interview. More information may be needed or the condition may appear serious or the outcome doubtful. At this stage, support is usually more important than blithe or premature reassurance. The doctor would do well to make clear that he appreciates how the patient must feel and that he will be in a better position to provide more definitive information once all the remaining investigations and outstanding information have been assessed.

Some patients may deny that they are ill or need help. There are patients who ignore medical advice and prefer to follow their own inclinations. Confronting such a patient with his denial or defensiveness can help bring about a more realistic discussion.

Throughout the consultation, the doctor's professionalism, competence and credibility are being scrutinized by the patient. Every interview is therefore an opportunity for strengthening the patient's faith in the doctor and compliance. Conversely, a poor interview style can seriously jeopardize the development of the patient's confidence and faith.

PROBLEM SITUATIONS

The doctor–patient relationship tends to elicit attitudes and behaviour which reflect previous relationships with figures in authority including other doctors, teachers or parents. The more sick, helpless and vulnerable the patient feels, the more likely his behaviour will reflect these attitudes. For example, a patient who has had an ambivalent and competitive relationship with his father may react to the doctor in the same way even though the doctor has done nothing to provoke such a reaction. Thus the interaction between doctor and patient can become highly charged with emotion and this in turn can seriously affect the behaviour of both doctor and patient. Some of the commoner responses that cause problems for the doctor include silence, overtalkativeness, evasiveness, seductiveness, suspicion, anger and aggressive behaviour, and passive or dependent behaviour.

The silent patient

Many doctors feel uncomfortable with a silent patient. The clinician usually feels that there is a task to be performed and that silence on the patient's part wastes precious time. Thus silence can provoke anger or irritation on the part of the doctor. However, with practice doctors can usually learn to permit a reasonable amount of silence to elapse by which time most patients will speak.

It is important for the doctor to establish whether the patient is seriously depressed which may account for the silence. There may be a need to question the patient about symptoms of depression as well as search for the classic verbal and non-verbal signs of depression (e.g. the patient's expression, posture, attitudes, behaviour) in order to clarify the diagnosis.

Silence at other times during an interview may indicate considerable emotion on the part of the patient, a need for time to think or reluctance or embarrassment. The doctor may help break the silence by repeating the last question or indeed the patient's last response or by indicating that perhaps the patient feels anxious or shy or a little fearful of talking further. Acknowledging that it can in certain circumstances be difficult to put things into words often helps ease the situation for the patient.

The overtalkative patient

The doctor has to learn how to keep the interview focused even when the patient is pedantic, circumstantial or overinclusive. A valuable interview skill is how to interrupt politely and appropriately. Certain phrases help, e.g. 'Let us come back to that point but can I just clarify something we touched on earlier . . .'; 'I can see that's important but first tell me . . .'; 'We will come to that later but first it would help me if I could be clear about . . .'. If the patient believes that whatever he has just touched on will at some later stage be considered he/she is usually quite happy to be directed according to the doctor's own consultation agenda.

Some patients ramble discursively. The doctor must gain control even if it means interrupting repeatedly and asking direct questions. Obsessional patients insist on providing extensive and redundant detail. Once again, the doctor can usually gain control by repeatedly pointing out that initially the simple facts are required and the detail can come later. Some patients talk continuously and rapidly because they are anxious. A friendly and supportive comment about the patient's evident anxiety is often sufficient to reduce it.

The angry patient

Some people become bad-tempered and irritable when ill. They can be angry, demanding and highly critical of everyone they encounter. Sometimes this reflects considerable anxiety. Sometimes it reflects resentment about depending on others. If the doctor responds with anger, this will damage the relationship and reduces the possibility of helping the patient further. When a patient becomes angry during a consultation or is angry from the outset it is useful if the doctor tries to calmly examine what is happening. Acknowledging that the patient is angry and asking him or her to explain why can be helpful.

In other circumstances the doctor may find himself the target of anger which is totally unconnected with him. For some reason, the patient may have been prevented from exhibiting his frustration and anger appropriately and displaces these feelings onto the doctor. In time the anger usually subsides. Once again, acknowledging the anger and making it plain that the source of the anger is unclear usually leads the patient to calm down a little and reveal what is the matter.

The evasive patient

When a patient shows evidence of evasiveness, it is a mistake to react by asking more detailed, specific and precise questions as this may cause the patient to become more embarrassed or uncomfortable. Instead, it is best to enquire directly about the patient's unease and discomfort. A comment such as 'You seem to find this difficult to talk about ...', or 'I sense you are not finding this easy ...' often enables the patient to indicate what is going on. After such a discussion it should be easier for the enquiry to continue.

GENERAL POINTS

Most of the problems that surround the consultation can be eased if attention is paid to some basic points. The position adopted by the doctor vis-à-vis the patient, for example, is important. Face-to-face meetings across a table are often perceived as more competitive and confrontational than seating arrangements which have doctor and patient sitting at right angles, perhaps across the corner of a table. Distance between doctor and patient is also important. Too close suggests intrusion of body space and therefore threat; too distant suggests coolness and uninvolvement. There are often cultural differences in relation to body space and these can lead to misunderstanding.

Certain postures, such as leaning forward from time to time, head nodding and maintaining a reasonable amount of eye-to-eye contact help patients see their doctors as warm, empathic and involved. Conversely, if the doctor does not look interested, maintains poor eye contact or maintains a formal and detached manner, patients may find it difficult to discuss intimate matters or to relax and communicate freely and effectively. But sometimes too intense eye contact can deter patients from talking freely and experience suggests that the doctor busying himself with some aspect of the physical examination can enable the patient to talk about an embarrassing matter, e.g. a sexual worry, which would otherwise be difficult to express.

SUGGESTED FURTHER READING

Byrne, P.S. and Long, B.E.L. (1976) *Doctors Talking to Patients*, London: HMSO.
Institute of Psychiatry (1978) *Notes on Eliciting and Recording Clinical Information*, Oxford: Oxford University Press.
Pendleton, D. and Hasler, J. (1983) *Doctor–Patient Communication*, London: Academic Press.

Chapter 4

Providing relevant information for patients and their families

Jenifer Wilson-Barnett

Relevant information can serve as a vital resource for those who are unwell. Unfortunately, members of the health care professions often seem unable to satisfy this need. There are many reasons for this and much to learn about why information is important and the best ways in which it can be provided. Essentially, staff must realize that information-giving is but one element in the process of communication. Information will only benefit those who want it, when they accept this need, in the form they appreciate. In the past, despite attempts to provide information by staff, there has possibly been too little attention to assessment of need by those trying to cope with illness. This chapter aims to demonstrate the importance of information-giving and provide guidelines for practitioners. It emphasizes this process in the context of hospital care because of evidence that this is a stressful environment and patients' information needs are maximized. However, the principles involved in assessing the need for, and providing, information, are relevant to all health care practice.

INFORMATION-GIVING IN THE CONTEXT OF HEALTH CARE

Increasingly 'self-care' or 'lay care' is being seen as ideal for those coping with ill-health in the acute or chronic situation. Independence rather than dependence is thought to encourage recovery or a better utility of life. This means that the style of health service provision is also changing. Rather than a pattern of 'caring for', nurses, doctors and others are trying to provide patients and their relatives with the strengths, knowledge and skills to care for themselves, in the longer term. This orientation implies the necessity of collaboration and negotiated plans of care, rather than professional prescription and advice-giving and assumed consent. Of course, for some patients this will not be possible – either not relevant or desirable – but members of staff should certainly never assume this to be the case without very careful consideration of the wishes of individuals concerned, the degree of infirmity and the agreed goals of treatment.

This re-orientation is reflective of the current value being placed on individual autonomy and a realization that patterns of illness are also changing. Although acute or emergency treatments are still required, more people suffer from chronically disabling conditions and these patients have the time to seek out information and weigh up alternatives. Fewer people are unquestioning and they usually wish to be fully consulted when in receipt of the health care services. Despite this tide of change, some professional staff have been slow to respond and it is salutary, but necessary, to review the evidence of the inadequacy of information-giving and open communication in health care.

BUREAUCRACY AND HEALTH CARE: BLOCKS TO INFORMATION EXCHANGE

The setting or environment of organized health care often seems to mitigate against open communication and access to information for clients. More recently, concentration of resources in large centres and hospitals is seen as necessary for reasons of economic efficiency and for provision of expertise across an increasingly expanding range of medical services and specialities. As a consequence, there has been an exponential growth in the size of organizations devoted to health care. On entry, individuals seeking help are usually exposed to various 'registering' procedures and received by lay personnel responsible for records and appointments. Access to professional services is therefore controlled and restricted. This is conventional and usually expected, but it does tend to give an impression of depersonalization and distance between the client and doctors or other professionals.

Depending on the attitude and the social skills of the secretary/receptionist, potential patients may feel welcomed and relaxed, or tense and hesitant. When entering a primary care surgery or a clinic, the individual may feel apprehension about his condition, but he may be accompanied (a well-known buffer to stress) and the setting is usually familiar. Even so, many people forget what they wished to say and fail to recall what the doctor advised. This may be a reflection of anxiety and a lack of real opportunities to communicate openly, in part, because of workload pressures.

In hospital, the atmosphere may reinforce the impression that the system is depersonalizing. Much information is required from patients and they may feel rather exhausted and overwhelmed by all that is happening. Patients report that staff are friendly, but they also realize that they are extremely busy and short of time.

It is in these contexts that research studies have described the inadequacy of communications and report a lack of information being provided for the recipients of care. Opinion surveys over the last twenty years show that a varying but substantial proportion of recipients are dissatisfied with the information they were given. For hospitalized patients in particular, many problems and complaints were found to be due to poor or incomprehensible information being provided on treatments and after care. Relatives and patients tended to feel they were not forewarned about events or prepared for life at home. This had caused distress when they were relatively isolated from health care staff, with fewer opportunities to ask questions.

There is some indication that the situation may be improving, smaller proportions of respondents being critical of information given to them. However, the rapid 'turnover' and admission rates in hospital attest to increasing pressures on the service and preparing people for discharge home is becoming more important, as more of the recovery process will be occurring outside the hospital. At the time of admission and discharge, so much information is required by patients and their friends.

Many may puzzle over why patients and their family members do not take more assertive action and request more information. Of course, many people do ask and receive desired information, and there are others who do not feel the need for additional information other than that which staff offer. However, there are explanations as to why a persistent group of patients remain dissatisfied, yet do not ask for more information.

In one study an over-riding feeling of gratitude and not wishing to trouble staff was found to be characteristic of patients, who also felt that it was really only appropriate to discuss care which concerned their physical recovery. They felt that staff did not encourage or welcome questions or requests for psychological support. It may therefore be the non-verbal communication of staff which provides a clear message to those they care for. The hustle and spread of movement in a clinic or ward may indicate that there are many tasks to be completed and interruptions are unwelcome. Facial expressions and body posture (turning away) may also deter patients or relatives from asking for information.

Anxiety and fatigue for patients being either diagnosed or treated may also be deterrents to normal confident behaviour. Not only do these feelings reduce initiative, but they may also be distracting, rendering the individual unable to formulate plans and think logically. Thus, they may feel unable to understand information if it were offered to them. Alternatively, they may be too afraid to ask for information which could lead on to unwanted disclosures and discussion.

WHY INFORMATION IS NECESSARY

Uncertainty and ignorance (rather than being blissful) are often distressing. Individuals need to make sure of their situation and in order to do this they may require additional information. Patients in particular need to interpret events in order to feel in control of their lives as much as possible. To some small degree people can tolerate unpredictable and unfamiliar occurrences, but major illness may reduce all certainty and leave a bewildered, helpless person. Further strange and threatening events may render them totally unable to cope and deeply depressed. Helplessness and 'lack of control' must be avoided as they may induce permanent psychological morbidity.

In order to prevent health care becoming threatening and unsupportive, information to individuals on what is happening and what is going to happen is essential. All staff should try to maintain or restore a sense of a person's self-control. At times of maximum uncertainty information needs are vital. However, anxiety may also be at a peak and information may not be processed effectively. Staff should therefore plan to provide this help beforehand so that recipients can understand what will occur, plan how they will cope and tolerate any discomfort involved without undue distress.

STRESSFUL EVENTS: INFORMATION NEEDS

Admission to hospital

Several studies have demonstrated that specific information on admission to hospital reduces anxiety and the harmful physical correlates of this emotion which complicate recovery. It has been the initiatives to help children cope with hospital that have provided such an excellent example for others. Information about the ward, the staff, the operation and visiting arrangements has been packaged in various ways for children. Cartoons, puppet shows, photographs and picture books were all found to help youngsters be more prepared for their stay. Such research found that pictures should include children as patients and that the use of participative games before admission prevented distress for both the child and the parents. The National Association for the Welfare of Children in Hospital has produced several booklets of this kind.

Adults are also found to experience more anxiety at the beginning of their hospital stay, before they become adjusted. Interview studies have typically found patients talking about their fear of the unknown and this points to their need for prior knowledge. Unfortunately, over half the patients admitted do not receive the standard hospital admission booklet (Moores and Thompson 1986). Booklets vary in quality, but provide a good opportunity to give information beforehand, at a time when patients can think about their plans and coping strategies.

Face-to-face information exchange for newly admitted patients

It is difficult to provide relevant information without asking people what they want to know and trying to understand their perspective. For newly admitted patients it is very important to use open communication and establishing a rapport is an important pre-condition to information exchange. They require orientation to the physical geography of the ward, particularly the bathroom area, and the names of staff involved in their care. If the staff member receiving them asks about their reactions to coming into hospital or their major concerns, they may feel more supported and appropriate information can be imparted. Clerical and routine information needs of the ward should be considered secondary to providing comfort and reassurance.

An account of future events in a chronological order will probably be appreciated at this time. Where possible, it is useful to include relatives or close friends in this conversation. As some of this information may be forgotten by the patient who is probably anxious, another person may helpfully remind them and talk over what is going to happen. The comfort received from a 'significant other' can be substantial and on no account should staff attempt to isolate the patient by waiting until such visitors have left the ward.

Discussion about the individual's condition and treatment may follow on after giving general information about the ward and sequence of events after being admitted into hospital. Adults will have some ideas and a varying amount of knowledge about their illness and possible treatment. It is wise to explore their understanding prior to talking about likely approaches. As the history unfolds, misconceptions or concerns can be noted and a plan for providing clear and correct information should be devised. Such information may be supplied immediately if the matter is straightforward and treatment imminent. Careful consideration should be given as to when best to discuss sensitive topics such as the state of a tumour, and other team members should be included.

It is important to realize that the first days in hospital will be anxiety-evoking for most patients, who may need information repeated. Also this early familiarization with staff may create a lasting impression of their priorities and attitudes to the patient. It is important to create the impression that one is willing to answer any questions whenever required.

Diagnostic tests: informing the patient

Undergoing diagnostic tests is found to cause extreme anxiety for a majority of individuals (such procedures as special X-rays, biopsies and scans are included in this category). Once more 'fear of the unknown' is mentioned most frequently, along with the underlying fear of the diagnostic revelation. It is also quite clear that insufficient information is provided by staff for the needs of patients. All too frequently tests are seen as 'routine', although patients may be completely unaware of what is involved. Despite extensive research which demonstrates the benefits of careful pre-test information on the purpose, procedure and sensations involved, neither in- nor out-patients systematically receive this.

The type of information found to be most useful includes details of greatest relevance and meaning to patients, such as:

1   The name and purpose of the test.
2   Time it will take to do the procedure.
3   When it will be carried out.
4   What preparation is required (e.g. starvation, bowel preparation).
5   Account of procedure including details of anaesthetic and analesia.
6   Sensations involved (e.g. pressure, bloating).
7   Guidance on coping with sensations.
8   After effects (if any).
9   When the results will be available.

Such information can be given verbally or in writing, or both, but with very careful thought given to the vocabulary used. It is extremely difficult for staff and students to use non-technical terms which are readily understood by non-medical people. It is important to give information on how discomfort can be minimized. Patients should always be encouraged to relate any pain they experience and request further pain-killing medication or sedation.

This type of information should be given at a time when the individual is alert and, hope-fully, not too anxious. It should be imparted interactively and, where a written paper has been prepared, this should be used in conjunction with conversation. Most essentially this discussion should commence with questions to the patient on what they particularly want to know and whether they have any concerns or worries. Few can retain other information which seems unimportant if they have a burning issue they wish to discuss.

The purpose of this information is to provide a 'cognitive map' of events for the patient.

This information should be given well before a major test. Usually this occurs at a time when consent is requested, the evening before the test. Ideally this interval should provide the patient with the opportunity to reflect on the information, read through the leaflet (if there is one) and ask for clarification if necessary. The aim is to provide a realistic account so that the anticipated and actual experiences correspond as much as possible. This should help people to feel more prepared for and less frightened by any unanticipated occurrences. Discomfort is also much easier to tolerate if the likely duration for this is established.

Results of tests should always be revealed to patients conscientiously. Too often N.A.D. (nothing abnormal discovered) results are filed as routine and not reported back to patients, who may be anxiously awaiting these.

Surgery: providing preparatory information

Fears associated with a surgical operation are often very deeply held: effects of the anaesthetic, the severity of pain, of being cut and 'what will they find?' being the most common. As high anxiety is correlated with longer and more complicated recovery patterns, it is essential that information is tailored to the specific needs of individual patients and that attention to their responses determines the course of the discussion.

Some details of surgery are usually provided by staff in the out-patient department and then this may be reinforced or elaborated by the general practitioner or others in the community. It is essential to gain an understanding of the patient and also their next of kin's views on the surgery, on what will be done and how long recovery will take. Further details can help them build on this and be less confusing for them.

Obviously decisions about whether to undergo surgery have been made by the time of hospitalization. Worries may well have been aired with the general practitioner and much of the preparatory information on surgery digested. It is therefore important to individualize the process of psychological preparation, although general principles may apply. A chronological account of what will occur and what will be done is usually provided to some extent when the consent form is signed. Explanation at this time is concerned with ensuring that the patient, and possibly the next of kin, understands the effects of surgery and how this will treat their problems. It is useful if another member of staff is involved (as an observer) in order to help clarify any points later or repeat what has been said.

More general information on ward-based events, or after-care and pain control, may be provided by nursing or other medical staff. However, this must be done considerately and sometimes only the minimum of information can be provided, or else there will be overload. Choosing what is most important for the patient and presenting this slowly and clearly is necessary.

One of the greatest skills in information-giving is selecting those facts which are most meaningful or useful to the recipient. Instructions for post-operative exercises and pain control are particularly important, as are explanations for the presence of dressings, drips and drains. Without forewarning these may be greeted with surprise and sometimes with terror. Lack of interest or signs of fatigue and anxiety should provide a clue as to the usefulness of the information. Interrupting the conversation for a short break or asking whether there is something else they wish to discuss seems to be a good ploy.

One rather important yet difficult issue to be discussed with surgical patients relates to questions about the risks of surgery. Surgeons constantly review chances for some advanced techniques and study the odds for advanced conditions. It is frequently impossible to give accurate figures and only approximations can be offered. Providing these details requires a background of wisdom in this area and other staff should learn to be quite honest if they cannot supply this or other types of information adequately.

Summary guidelines are provided below using elements of interventions which have been shown to be beneficial for patients prior to special tests or surgery.

1   Sessions should be interactive but provide a chronological account of the procedure and its efforts.
2   Major queries or concerns should be explored initially.
3   All information should be given in everyday language.
4   Patients should be encouraged to ask questions and write things down if they wish.
5   A written account can be used to guide the session and left with the patient for future reference.
6   Information which relates to the patient's experience and sensations is most important.
7   Advice on physical coping is particularly useful if the patient is conscious during a procedure.
8   The patient should be constantly assessed for signs of fatigue or fear.
9   If information does not appear to be relevant to the patient a different approach should be tried, e.g. exercises or relaxation.

Patients who do not wish to know

There are a small number of people who do not wish for information about a stressful event as a resource to help them cope. It is essential to establish a good rapport with such patients to ensure that they can express their wishes openly. In any approach patients must be given a choice as to whether they are provided with information. Some may prefer to use a different strategy such as diversion and denial. There is some evidence to suggest that information may be unhelpful and even harmful to these individuals. Their lack of anxiety puts them in a good state to recover, as long as they are motivated to act positively and do not become resentful about the discomfort.

Pre-operative information prior to admission

Written information for pre-operative patients has also been produced and may serve as a valuable asset when this can be studied prior to admission. It does seem, however, that there may be several advantages to providing them with pre-operative classes as out-patients, as long as patients are really given a choice as to whether they attend or not. Such a group might be able to share concerns and gain a realistic and positive appraisal of the pre-operative period. Ideally, staff from the surgical ward(s) might meet patients to promote continuity of care.

So often, however, surgery is performed without much notice and patients may be

suffering physical pain when they are admitted. Close contact and a gentle and more oppor-
tunistic style of information giving is then required.

INFORMATION REQUIRED FOR RECOVERY

Coping with recovery or trying to optimize one's health potential after long-term illness
requires great effort. Many factors influence recovery and one of the greatest is the knowledge and skill base of the patient and family members. Although this type of information-
giving has been described as patient-teaching, patients and their families often have great
wisdom and understanding about illness and treatment to give to staff. So, once more it is
obvious that assessment of need is fundamental to planning this process. Participants need to
feel at ease with one another and have mutual respect for their abilities and wishes.

Teaching for recovery at home may commence in hospital in the ward or clinic after diagnosis or treatment. However, there is evidence that this is unsystematic, although there are
notable exceptions in specialized areas such as cardiac and cancer centres. However, those
recovering from surgery or a coronary thrombosis, those adjusting to a long-term condition
such as diabetes or rheumatism or those newly diagnosed as suffering from cancer have
much to learn and master. Helping them is challenging and difficult.

Planning and assigning this function to specific staff is a prerequisite to its successful
implementation. Scheduling 'sessions' in advance when relatives can also attend and registering this on the care plan adds to the commitment. As this is a complex area, several
sessions may be required. Nurses, physiotherapists, doctors and dietitians may be included
or asked for advice when necessary. Emotional or sensitive topics may be covered and staff
members should be well-informed and confident. At times this process may adopt the style
and forms of counselling. However, many families and individuals appreciate more information on what they can do to maximize their health.

Teaching should be based on an agreed plan with patients and their spouse or family
members. It cannot be successful if it is not accepted as necessary by them, or if individuals
are too emotionally upset to think of the future. Assessment of the patients' readiness,
previous knowledge and experiences of illness is therefore required initially. The first session
may well explore their view of the illness and ideas about recovery or adjustment. This
discussion may help to clarify thinking and identify areas of need for information or skills.

Goals should be set for 'teaching sessions' together so that there is mutual understanding.
Relatives may have additional needs and these should of course be recognized. Usual information includes guidelines on diet, activity, minor symptoms that might be predicted and the
sort of treatment plan envisaged.

Sessions should be assigned topics and a realistic timetable agreed. For those in hospital,
prior to discharge, two or three sessions may be feasible. Issues of major concern should be
tackled first and each session should commence with a reiteration of the goals and a brief
summary of what was covered previously. Information should be provided in an interactive
informal style and should aim to be enjoyable. No more than three topics should be discussed
in a single session, which should usually last no more than twenty minutes.

'Teaching' in a person's home, or a doctor's office, is often so much easier than in a busy
hospital ward, as a quiet, undisturbed environment is desirable. Everybody involved should

be comfortably seated and relaxed. Materials to illustrate the session and equipment required should be collected first to avoid subsequent interruptions. Illustrations are particularly useful to explain surgical techniques, such as hysterectomy, or for younger patients in order to hold their interest. When skills need to be taught, such as blood pressure measurement, injections or the application of dressings, demonstrations should adapt to the facilities that will be available in the domestic setting, rather than those of the ready-made hospital treatment room. Subjects should be permitted to handle equipment and experiment with different methods.

Leaflets which prescribe exact times for resuming certain activities are sometimes unhelpful. For if patients do not wish to resume activities at the specified time, they may feel inadequate or worried and, on the other hand, those who are ready sooner may hold back unnecessarily.

Reiteration of information can indicate the success of sessions and degree of understanding. A tactful way to ask for this is, 'Mr Jones, can you just tell me what you thought we talked about last time?', or, 'Mr Jones, can you just show me which technique we decided on for your injection?'. However, in the final evaluation, it is the extent to which the process results in good recovery or adjustment which is most important. Health carers themselves may also evaluate their performance, by the extent to which they listened to the patient, gave accurate and useful information, searched for the facts they did not know and the degree of satisfaction the participants reported.

Leaflets for discharged patients

Some information can be provided in a standardized way, but those leaflets which allow for individualized comments or particular plans are most useful. Prescribing details and medical advice may be written on a continuity or cooperation card for the use of patients, their family and other staff involved in their care and these certainly serve as a reminder for all concerned, particularly if drug regimes are complex and varied on different days of the week.

Specific recovery booklets which provide generalized information for those with a particular condition (cardiac, gynaecological) are also sometimes helpful. They can be used to augment and focus discussion or information exchange. It is even more helpful where an individual's exercise and diet plans are incorporated on blank pages. Goals reached can be ticked off and this may provide a psychological lift for the patient and family.

SUMMARY

From the previous sections in this chapter, it must be clear that information-giving is an important and challenging aspect of care. Professionals can no longer prescribe or advise and automatically expect patients to obey or comply. Assessment of wishes and need is therefore essential prior to giving information.

In summary, certain key points to health carers can be identified:

1   Be sure of the purpose for information-giving.
2   Be clear about the outcome for this.

3   Consider the most important items of information required to achieve this and note these on paper.
4   Clarify that these are needed by the subject.
5   Consider the accuracy of the information – check the facts.
6   Practise information-giving with peers before engaging in this with patients – eliminate technical terms.
7   Always ask what information the subject would prefer.
8   Try to appear relaxed and confident.
9   Ask if the client's spouse is comfortable or in need of anything.
10   Ask if they have immediate, or burning questions and, if so, tackle these first.
11   Agree a structure on topics for information.
12   Encourage interaction.
13   Listen well and leave silences to promote comment or questions.
14   Try to help subjects enjoy the conversation.
15   Do not avoid emotive issues, but always ask patients if these should be explored.
16   Never overload with information. Remember those who are ill, elderly or nervous cannot tolerate much information at one time.
17   Write notes as aide-mémoire for the subjects.
18   On concluding a conversation, briefly recapitulate on the topics covered and ask for further issues to be discussed at a future time.
19   Participation by patients and relatives is essential if they are to use the information.
20   Evaluation by reiteration and demonstration by subjects is most meaningful but must be done tactfully.
21   Be self-questioning as to how this might have been more sensitively or effectively done.

Planning information-giving

A systematic approach to information-giving is required so that all those who wish for this actually receive it. This implies that it should be noted down on care plans or case notes and other documents which help to direct care. American agencies insist on this type of written record for billing purposes, but in the United Kingdom it may stimulate a certain redirection to care, where psychological needs are given the same priority as physical care.

A team approach

Collaboration between medical and other staff in this process should avoid problems of over-lapping authority or a conflict in the type of information given. Opportunities for the team to discuss information needs and resources for this should not be missed. Records of information-giving should be kept for all to review. The care plan, or cooperation card, is an ideal vehicle for this as the patient and his family also have full access to this. They can then comment on all care received and needed. This sharing of information exchange is even more important when sensitive issues are broached. For instance, requests for full information on diagnosis or prognosis should certainly be noted down.

Concluding remarks

Skills required to become a good 'informer' are similar to those needed for good communications. However, acquisition of these complex skills sometimes takes substantial training and feedback, something which has not been recognized or supported in the past. The art of being sensitive to others' needs, establishing a rapport, picking up cues and asking open questions appropriately is necessary to providing relevant and requested information. Staff need to learn to see things from the patient's or family's perspective and empathize with their needs. However, professionals are unlikely to succeed in this role unless they ask questions, listen to the answers, seek out information and constantly update their own communication practice.

SUGGESTED FURTHER READING

Johnson, J.E. (1983) 'Preparing patients to cope with stress while hospitalised', in J. Wilson-Barnett (ed.) *Patient Teaching*, Edinburgh: Churchill Livingstone, pp. 19–23.

Klug-Redman, B. (1981) *Issues and Concepts in Patient Education*, New York: Appleton Century-Croft.

Moores, B. and Thompson, A.G.H. (1986) 'What 1357 hospital patients think about aspects of their stay in British acute hospitals', *Journal of Advanced Nursing* 11: 87–102.

Wilson-Barnett, J. (ed.) (1983) *Patient Teaching*, Edinburgh: Churchill Livingstone.

Wilson-Barnett, J. (1989a) 'Limited autonomy and partnership: professional relationships in health care', *Journal of Medical Ethics* 15: 1, 12–16.

Wilson-Barnett, J. (1989b) 'Distressing hospital procedures', in T. Byrne and H. Lacey (eds) *Psychological Management of the Physically Ill*, Edinburgh: Churchill Livingstone, pp. 300–15.

Wilson-Barnett, J. and Fordham, M. (1982) *Recovery From Illness*, Chichester: John Wiley & Sons.

Part II

Developing specific communication and counselling skills

Chapter 5

Identifying emotional and psychosocial problems

Linda Gask

PATIENTS PRESENT WITH PROBLEMS

Patients don't go to see their doctor with a diagnosis but with a problem. The man who has occasional chest pain on exertion will be unlikely to complain of angina *per se* but will tell you that he is very worried about the pain that he is having in his chest. Similarly, the woman who is having abdominal pain will not necessarily tell you that she is suffering from 'depression', but she may tell you perhaps that she has been very worried by the pains in her stomach and that she fears that she may have cancer. We are trained to seize upon these presenting symptoms and arrive at the 'correct' diagnosis (I have used quotation marks because this is often wrongly taken only to mean a physical diagnosis, with a psychological diagnosis merely being arrived at by exclusion), but in doing this we may fail to understand what the patient sees as the main reason for consulting or what he sees his problems to be.

Key tasks

Much of the teaching that we receive centres on how to ask the checklist of questions that will enable us to arrive at a diagnosis, either psychological or physical. However, if we begin to test out our hypotheses about what the diagnosis may be very early in a consultation, by asking too many closed questions (these are questions to which the patient can only answer yes or no, such as 'Have you had any pain in your back?' or 'Have you been sleeping well?') we risk failing to achieve the other major tasks of the consultation. These are:

1   To identify what are the patient's main symptoms and what worries them about their symptoms. We need to know why this person has come now with this particular

complaint, what they fear it may be and also what their expectations of treatment are.

2   To identify any important psychosocial problems which may have a bearing on both what the patient is worried about and whether they will be able to comply with treatment.

3   To identify illness, both physical and/or psychological. Psychological illness may not be immediately apparent from the patient's presenting complaints.

The majority of patients with new psychological illness who visit their general practitioner present with physical symptoms. We call this phenomenon somatization. The reasons for this are several. First, the patient may think that the doctor expects him or her to produce physical symptoms. Somatic symptoms feature in the presenting symptoms of depression and anxiety but the patient may choose the somatic symptoms to justify a visit to the doctor. Second, symptoms that the patient has had for a long time, such as a pain, may seem worse during an episode of depression, so these are presented to the doctor. Third, patients who are anxious or depressed commonly notice bodily sensations more than they usually would and finally there is the stigma of mental illness which should not be underestimated. By our tendency to diagnose psychological illness only by exclusion we may confirm our patients' beliefs that it isn't acceptable to complain of depression.

Using skills

So what skills are needed to ensure that we can carry out these tasks? There are simple things that can be said and done in interviews that will ensure that patients have the opportunity to express their concerns and worries and talk about how they feel. All these skills can and should be used by all those who work in the caring professions including doctors, nurses, occupational therapists, physiotherapists and social workers. So although most of the examples shown here are of doctor/patient interactions the word 'doctor' can be taken to represent any health professional. The pronoun 'he' has been used for both doctor and patient throughout for the purposes of simplicity only.

We shall consider first how to get started, then look at the basic skills of listening, watching and feeling, followed by how to respond to cues and demonstrate empathy. There are occasions when screening questions for psychological symptoms are helpful and we shall look at these and choose ones that may be particularly useful.

Examples are provided in each section, and a short excerpt from an interview is included to give a feel for how these interventions fit together.

Getting started

Whenever you are talking to patients, try and ensure that you have somewhere private to interview them. This will help the patient to feel comfortable enough to talk about feelings and worries without fear of being overheard.

Ensure that you start the interview well. Introduce yourself, mention the patient's name and follow this up with a clear, open-ended question such as 'What can I do for you?' or 'How are you?' At this point it's essential to look at the patient and make eye-contact. He will then feel that you are ready to listen to him. Don't start writing immediately and if you want to make notes or glance at case notes ask the patient's permission to do this first, otherwise he will be unsure whether or not to carry on talking. If you are a student you should discuss with the patient what will happen to any notes that you make. In certain situations, where your task is to assess the patient's problems and you have limited time, you should tell the patient exactly how much time you have. This will then make it easier for you to control the interview later if necessary (see p. 44).

If you are interrupted by the phone, or someone coming into the room, ask the patient's permission to deal with the interruption. When you are alone with the patient again, or your conversation on the telephone is over, summarize where you were up to before the interruption, for example: 'Now you were saying just a moment ago that . . .'

This will demonstrate that your attention is again with the patient and will help to convey your interest.

BASIC SKILLS

Once the interview has begun the three basic skills required are to be able to listen, to watch and to be aware of your own feelings, because these are the three main sources of information at your disposal.

Listening

What the patient says is an obvious indicator to what is worrying them or how they are feeling. Frequently people use words which may provide us with a clue as to how they are feeling. We call these words or statements verbal cues. Examples might be 'I'm really fed up with it all . . .' or 'It's really getting me down . . .'. Ways in which these cues can be responded to are described below.

Watching

Patients may do certain things which are an important clue to how they feel, or they may use a particular tone of voice when they talk about something which worries them. We call these non-verbal and vocal cues. Responding to such cues may also be very helpful in detecting what the patient is worried about.

Feeling

Notice how you feel yourself when you are talking to someone. Patients generate all sorts of feelings in us and by identifying how we feel we may realize the impact that such a patient has on friends and family. This can help us to understand our patients' circumstances more clearly.

Responding to cues

You can respond to patient's verbal cues in three different ways:

1 By asking an open question, for example:
Patient: I've been feeling very out of sorts recently.
Doctor: Mmm . . . How have you been feeling?
If you can't ask this immediately, make a mental note and return to it:
Doctor: You said a moment ago that you had been feeling 'out of sorts' . . . how have you been feeling?

2 By clarifying what has been said, e.g.:
Doctor: What do you mean when you say 'out of sorts?'
In this way you get the patient to say what they mean when they use a particular word. Remember that you may not understand quite the same by a particular medically loaded word such as 'panic' or 'depression' as the patient does.

3 By asking for an example:
Nurse: When was the last time that you felt like that? Can you tell me about it?
Patient: Well, I think it was when I was out at the shops yesterday.
Nurse: Can you tell me what actually happened?

This is a particularly useful way of obtaining a lot of information very quickly, and enables you to understand exactly what is happening. It can also throw up quite a lot of other clues about the problems that patients may be experiencing which can then be further explored with more open questions and clarification. In fact a combination of these three interventions will provide you with a great deal of information without your having to guess and ask a lot of screening questions (such as 'Are things all right at work?' 'Have you any money worries?' and so on.). It isn't necessarily wrong to ask about such areas, it's simply that you will get there faster and get better information if you let the patient take you there himself. The patient will also feel that you are listening and are interested, because you respond to what he says.

As well as responding to verbal cues, you can also respond to non-verbal cues. This can be an exceptionally powerful way of getting patients to talk about feelings. A simple intervention with a tearful patient such as 'You look very upset at the moment' can give that person permission to talk about how they are feeling. Such statements often convey an understanding to the patient that you understand how they feel, and as such they demonstrate empathy. We shall explore this skill next.

Demonstrating empathy

Much of what is written about 'empathy' would tend to suggest that the conveying of it is something mystical and demands extensive training. In fact it's quite simple. You have to learn some straightforward ways of conveying to patients that you understand how it is for them and how they might be feeling given the situation they find themselves in. It differs from sympathy which isn't always helpful because it really means how you would feel if you found yourself in that situation, and giving sympathy may result in the patient feeling patronized rather than understood. To be empathic you have first to put yourself in the other person's shoes to understand how he feels and then show him that you are interested and understand. Sometimes we do the former without the latter. If you want to convey that understanding and interest you must:

1   Look at the patient, not all the time – which might be threatening – but certainly at key points such as when you ask the all important first question: 'What can I do for you?'
2   Tell the patient that you understand what is happening for them – e.g. 'I can see you've been having a really difficult time recently'.

Demonstrating empathy will enable you to build up a relationship with the patient in which a greater understanding of his or her problems will be achieved.

SOME IMPORTANT ADDITIONAL SKILLS

Asking about health beliefs and concerns

When a patient presents with physical symptoms, even if it seems apparent that there is no underlying psychological illness it is important to remember to ask what the patient thinks the symptoms are due to and if there is anything in particular that he is worried about. If you do this routinely you are much more likely to achieve patient compliance with treatment. However, there are other reasons why this is a useful technique. Patients with emotional illness may be preoccupied with fears of illness based on symptoms which they do not understand. These may be symptoms that they would otherwise not have noticed, symptoms of genuine physical illness or somatic symptoms of psychological illness. Whatever the cause, the patient's fears should be addressed. Such a question can provide the key to understanding what is going on when a patient presents with physical symptoms for which no clear organic cause can be found, but there is no other apparent evidence of psychological problems. Try and ask something like: 'Is there anything in particular that you have been worried about?'

Using the skills in practice

Doctor: You said a moment ago that you feel very tense. Can you say a little more about that?   **[Clarification]**

Patient: Well, I get very churned up, then my neck gets stiff and then the headache comes on (*change in tone of voice*).

Doctor: Umm . . . is there anything that you are particularly worried about with the headache? What have you thought it might be?   **[Health beliefs]**

Patient: I know it's silly . . . but I can't help thinking it might be a tumour. It's just like the sort of headache that my father had (*bursts into tears*).

Doctor: I can see you are very worried. **[Comment on non-verbal cue]** Would you like to say a little more about what happened to your father?　**[Empathic open question]**

Patient: I don't know ... I suppose we didn't always get on very well – he was a difficult man.

Doctor: What do you mean? **[Clarification]**

Patient: We argued all the time ... but I do miss him (*change in tone of voice*).

Doctor: I can see that you do. **[Empathic comment]**

Patient: And the last time we argued ... it was awful.

Doctor: Would you like to say what happened? **[Example]**

Patient: It was the week before he died ... I didn't know he was so ill. I thought he was just being his usual awkward self. We didn't know how serious the headaches were.

Maintaining appropriate control of the interview

By asking open questions, clarifying and seeking examples you should be able to keep the consultation flowing. 'Good' interviews (i.e. where patients are able to talk about their problems and feel satisfied afterwards) begin with the patient describing his symptoms and problems in his own words, move through a section where the doctor may ask about particular symptoms using screening questions (see below) and then on to a section where the doctor takes more control, gives information and negotiates a treatment contract with the patient. Occasionally patients give a great deal of information which is not directly relevant and they may need to be gently directed back to the question at hand. If you politely emphasize that what is being said is interesting and helpful, but you would like to return to what you had asked about a moment before, most patients will not be offended. They are much more offended by the doctor who rudely interrupts and appears not to be listening.

Patient: And then he said to me ...

Doctor: I wonder, would you mind if we returned to talking about that next time we meet? It's very helpful, but we only have a half hour today and I'd like just to return to what you meant when you said you were feeling 'down' yesterday.

SCREENING QUESTIONS

There are two occasions when you might want to ask questions that screen directly for emotional symptoms.

General screening questions

First, there are many interviews in which the patient does not present with any emotional symptoms, but as part of a general systems screen you will want to exclude the possibility of emotional problems. Why is it acceptable to ask about all the symptoms of cardiac or GI disease but not about emotional problems? Probably because we are concerned that we will antagonize patients by doing so. In fact there are some simple, non-threatening screening questions that should form part of any general systems review. These are:

How have you been sleeping?

How have you been eating?

Have you been feeling tired?

Have you felt particularly anxious?

Have you been worried about illness? (Discussed in further detail earlier.)

Have you been feeling low in spirits at all?

Most patients will not be unduly threatened by these questions (on the contrary they may be relieved that you have asked!) and the replies to them may provide important cues for you to follow up.

Screening for symptoms of depression and anxiety

This is something that you should do towards the end of any interview when you have talked about emotional difficulties and you have reason to suspect that your patient may be depressed and/or anxious to a degree that constitutes the onset of emotional illness. You can screen quickly for symptoms of major depression by asking about difficulty in sleeping, poor appetite, weight loss, concentration, interest, ideas of worthlessness, guilt and self blame and suicidal ideas. (Some patients who are depressed have increased sleep, appetite and weight.) Don't be afraid that by asking about suicide you will precipitate someone into action. Patients with such thoughts are again generally relieved to be able to share them. A quick screen for anxiety disorder should include questions about worrying, tension, restlessness, tension pains and physical symptoms of anxiety. It is beyond the scope of this chapter to talk in greater detail about symptoms of psychiatric illness, but remember to screen for additional symptoms that the patient may not have mentioned earlier. Don't do this too early in the interview, because you will take control prematurely and may prevent the patient from saying all that is on his mind. He may also feel that you are trying to label him with an illness (which some people will justifiably fear) and that you do not want to listen to him. Remember that many people do not perceive that severe emotional symptoms may constitute illness and you may have to sell this idea to them tactfully and gently.

IMPROVING YOUR SKILLS

The best way to do this is to try and record your interviews with patients and then watch them (or listen to them) either on your own or with colleagues. Many people use videotape for this purpose. That is fine if you have facilities that you can use; hospital departments of psychiatry and teaching departments of general practice and nursing have easy access to such facilities. Video is particularly good for helping you to notice non-verbal cues. Audio-recording can be just as useful though, and all you need is a domestic tape-recorder. However, if you have difficulty obtaining good sound you may find it is greatly improved by using an external microphone (such as the PZM flat microphone – obtainable from High Street electrical shops).

You must obtain the patient's informed consent before recording an interview, and explain the purpose, who it will be shown to and how it will be disposed of.

When you look at the interview, try and notice those points where you missed important cues, and keep stopping the tape to give yourself a chance to think how you might have handled something differently. Think also how you might have usefully employed some of the skills described above.

When you look at a tape in a group setting, there are several important things to remember:

1   Let the person who is showing the tape say something about the patient first, and encourage him to say what his difficulties were in the consultation, so that it is clear what he wants to get from the exercise.
2   Ensure that everyone knows that they can stop the tape at any time, but the person who does stop the tape is on the spot and must say what he would have done or said at that point in the interview to improve it.
3   Remember that to show others how you talk to patients is a risky business, and feelings can be easily hurt. Give positive feedback as well as providing criticism for each other. In that way, you will foster a safe atmosphere in which to learn, and it might even be enjoyable too!

SUMMARY

Patients present with problems. Identifying emotional and psychosocial problems involves using certain skills. Basic skills are Listening, Watching and Feeling. By using these skills you will learn to identify cues. There are a number of ways in which you can respond to verbal and non-verbal cues. Showing empathy will help you in your task. Additional important skills are learning how to control the interview and how to ask about health beliefs and concerns. Remember the screening questions that can be asked in any interview to screen for emotional problems, or can be asked at the end of an interview to help identify particular syndromes.

Give yourself the best possible chance by respecting the patient's privacy and confidentiality when you interview him, and this is especially important if you wish to record the interview.

SUGGESTED FURTHER READING

The following short list provides a background to the ideas expressed above:

Lesser, A.L. (1985) 'Problems based interviewing in general practice', *Medical Education* 19: 299–304.
Neighbour, R. (1987) *The Inner Consultation*, Lancaster: MTP Press.
Pendleton, D., Schofield, T., Tate, P. and Havelock, P. (1984) *The Consultation: An approach to learning and teaching*, Oxford: OUP.
Tuckett, D., Boulton, M. and Olson, C. (1985) *Meetings Between Experts: an approach to sharing ideas in medical consultations*, London: Tavistock.

Chapter 6

Managing difficult communication tasks

Peter Maguire

There are a number of particularly difficult communication tasks which doctors have to carry out including breaking bad news of a serious illness, coping with denial or managing a patient's distress or anger. There are, however, a number of skills which can be learnt to help and support patients during these stressful situations.

BREAKING BAD NEWS

Checking awareness

When you take a history of a patient's physical or mental illness you should check what he thinks might be wrong by asking, for example, 'When you noticed you were bleeding from the back passage what did you think it might be due to?' The patient may then answer 'Oh, I thought it was just haemorrhoids', or 'I was worried that it could be cancer'. Alternatively, you might have asked 'When you noticed you were getting low-spirited, irritable and lacking in energy had you any idea what it might be?' The patient may have answered 'I thought I was having some kind of nervous breakdown'.

When your patient realizes that he has a serious illness proceed by asking 'Are there any other reasons why you think that?' This allows him to confirm that he is fully aware that he has a serious condition ('I have been losing weight, I am off my food, I have no energy, I am getting increasing pain in my abdomen, so I think it's got to be cancer'). The depressed patient may say 'I have felt upset and sad in the past but never to this extent. I just can't pull myself out of it, it's taken over. At times I feel so low I don't want to go on. I feel I am losing control. It has to be a nervous breakdown hasn't it?' You should then confirm that the patient's belief is correct ('You're right. It is cancer'; 'Yes, you are having a form of nervous breakdown') before establishing and working through the patient's resulting concerns as discussed later. Some patients will respond to the question 'Any other reasons you think that' by moving back to denial ('I'm just being silly. I know it isn't serious'). Their denial should be respected.

Giving bad news

When your questioning establishes that your patient has no idea that he is seriously ill you face a difficult task; how to help him change his perception from his being well to having a serious illness. You can do this by giving a warning to alert him that his condition is not so straightforward. You must then pause to allow your information to be assimilated and enable him to indicate whether he wishes to be given more information or prefers to leave matters there. If he signals a wish to proceed select a phrase that indicates the possibility of a serious condition but still allows him room for manoeuvre. This will give the patient another opportunity to opt out or move further towards facing the truth. So, try to work out beforehand a hierarchy of euphemisms that you might use. The following dialogue illustrates how bad news can be broken.

Doctor: I am afraid this 'nervous breakdown' doesn't look so straightforward.

Patient: What do you mean, doesn't look so straightforward?

Doctor: Well, as you know when I first saw you and talked to you I thought it might be a depressive illness which would respond quickly to treatment. Now I am not so sure.

Patient: What do you mean 'not so sure'?

Doctor: As you admitted the other day some other symptoms have developed. You'll remember that you told me you had begun to hear voices and that at times you felt people were trying to control you by beaming laser beams at you?

Patient: Yes.

Doctor: Because of these developments I am afraid this could be a more serious illness.

Patient: More serious?

Doctor: I think it could be a form of schizophrenia.

Patient: Oh no! Won't that be the finish of me?

The patient's responses indicated that he wished to be told the truth about his condition even though it upset him. Another patient might have responded differently.

Doctor: I am afraid that this ulcer of yours doesn't look so simple.

Patient: How do you mean 'doesn't look so simple?'

Doctor: When we put the gastroscope down to look at your ulcer, it looked more serious than I had thought.

Patient: That's all right, I'll leave the details to you. What are you going to do for me?

This patient elected to avoid the truth and put his future in the consultant's hands.

Managing distress and exploring concerns

When you confirm that a patient's awareness is correct he is bound to be upset. For there is no way you can soften bad news. Your key task now is to help him manage his distress. You can best do this by acknowledging that he is upset ('I can see you are very upset') and then asking 'Could you bear to tell me just what's making you so upset?' This will encourage him to identify his resultant concerns. It is important that you elicit all of these ('Have you any other concerns'?) before you attempt to offer reassurance, advice or information. If you succumb to the natural temptation of offering advice and information before you have elicited all his concerns, he will not be receptive to what you say. He will be preoccupied with his undisclosed concerned and associated emotions. By acknowledging his distress and eliciting all his concerns you can help him move from experiencing what seems to be an intolerable level of distress to his feeling that the situation can be managed to some extent. Thus, your dialogue might go as follows:

Doctor: I am sorry to have to confirm that you are right. You have a form of schizophrenia. Could you bear to tell me (negotiating to explore concerns) why you are so upset?

Patient: It was bad enough to think I was having a nervous breakdown. To know that I have schizophrenia is too much to bear.

Doctor: Why do you feel that way? (clarification)

Patient: I have heard that it is an illness that you don't recover from and that it can destroy your personality. I am frightened that it will ruin my life.

Doctor: Do you have any other concerns about having schizophrenia? (screening)

Patient: I have heard that it can only be controlled by strong drugs. I am worried that I will need to be on drugs for the rest of my life. If that's the case I do not think that I want to go on living.

Doctor: Have you any other concerns? (screening)

Patient: Yes. I gather it can affect your capacity to feel.

Doctor: How do you mean? (clarification)

Patient: I gather some schizophrenics complain that they are no longer able to feel any emotion or be creative.

Doctor: That sounds important? (educated guess)

Patient: It is, I am an artist and my creativity is very important to me.

Doctor: Have you any other concerns? (screening)

Patient: No.

Now that you have established all his concerns, you should be able to foster an appropriate level of hope taking into account the likely prognosis. In this instance, you believe that he has a reasonable prognosis. So, you respond by saying 'While you do have a form of schizophrenia I think that it will respond reasonably quickly to treatment with appropriate medication. I am confident that you will recover. With regard to your needing to be on drugs for life, I think this is unlikely but, of course, I can only be sure of that over time. In the meantime the uncertainty about long-term drug treatment will be difficult for you. With regard to the effect of your illness on your ability to feel and create there isn't any problem with that at the moment is there? I see no reason why there should be.

By tackling each concern you will help the patient move from feeling that his life will be ruined to hoping that each of his concerns is resolvable in part, at least.

Once you have broken bad news, acknowledged distress, established and discussed resultant concerns and tried to resolve these you may be put under pressure to give information about the eventual outcome. It is vital that you tailor what you say to the likely outcome. Thus, faced with a patient with cancer appropriate statements might include 'I am sure we can eradicate it', 'I am sure we can control it for the time being', or 'I am hopeful we can ease your suffering'. If you offer false reassurance to patients and relatives they will feel bitter and betrayed when they realize that the information you gave them was incorrect and misleading. It also creates serious difficulties for colleagues who have to see the patient later.

When attempting to give an overall prognosis you should resist the temptation to provide a finite time. Predictions about the outcome of physical or mental illness are uncertain and doctors usually err on the side of optimism.

HANDLING UNCERTAINTY

When a patient asks 'Can I be cured?' or 'How long have I got'? the honest answer is the most difficult to give but the most helpful ('The problem is that I do not know'). You should then be empathic ('I guess that not knowing is hard for you'?) and allow the patient time to respond. Then explore his concerns by asking 'How does this leave you feeling?' You should then deal with any concerns you elicit as in the 'breaking bad news' sequence.

You still have the problem of how to help him live with this uncertainty. Begin by checking if he would like to be given any markers that would herald a progression of his illness ('Would you like me to give you some idea of what you might notice if your illness gets worse'?) Those patients who answer 'yes' should be given clear markers ('I think you would get very tired and breathless again and lose weight'). You should then point out that at the moment everything is under control – 'so as long as you don't have these symptoms you can tell yourself that you are alright ... and get on with your life'.

The patient should also be given a lifeline ('If at any stage you notice anything untoward do not hesitate to get in touch with me') and the frequency of assessment can then be nego-tiated. Few patients abuse this.

Doctor: I'd like to see you every two to three months from the medical viewpoint. But how often do *you* think you should be checked out?
Patient: Three months sounds a bit long. Can I make it two months and see how that goes?
Doctor: Sure.
Patient: I'm scared I'll go to pieces if it's left too long.
Doctor: O.K., we will make it every two months.

DIFFICULT QUESTIONS

When you face a difficult question like 'Have I got schizophrenia?' you should avoid false reassurance ('Of course you haven't, I am sure it's not schizophrenia') and explore why the patient is asking you this question.

Patient: Have I got schizophrenia?
Doctor: I *will* answer your question but it would help me if you could tell me why you are asking me.

Patient: I've been hearing voices. They keep saying horrible things about me and abusing me. I have heard from other people that people who hear voices have schizophrenia. I am also having trouble thinking straight. At times I even get the feeling that my thoughts are not my own and they are being imposed on me.

Doctor: Do you have any other reasons why you think you might have schizophrenia?

Patient: My father suffered from it and eventually killed himself. I am frightened that I am to end up like him.

Doctor: I can understand that. Are there any other reasons why you think you might have schizophrenia?

Patient: No.

Doctor: I have to tell you that you are right. You have put two and two together and it does make four. It looks as though you do have a schizophrenic illness.

When you reflected his question back this patient gave you good reasons for his question. Another patient may have said 'I know I am just being silly, I know it's not schizophrenia. It's some other kind of breakdown'. When this happens allow the patient to move into denial unless it hinders compliance with advice and treatment.

HANDLING DENIAL

When a patient denies the seriousness of his illness and his family are upset by this it is tempting to force him to confront reality. However, this may be harmful because patients usually only deny the reality of their predicament when it is too painful to face. Consequently, attempts to force them to do so can lead to serious psychiatric morbidity. Moreover, denial may be only a temporary defence until the patient feels ready to face what is happening. Consequently, you should be patient about denial instead of being confrontative. Even so, there are two ways you can use to test whether a patient is truly in denial or is ready to develop his awareness.

First, you can confront patients with key inconsistencies in their history which suggest that their conditions are serious rather than benign. For example, if you are faced with a woman who insists that her lump was benign but says that she had had a lumpectomy and a course of radiotherapy you can challenge her by saying 'I am puzzled that you say your lump was benign given that you have had a course of radiotherapy'. The woman may reply 'You may well be puzzled but I'm not, it doesn't worry me'. She does not wish to confront her reality and you should respect her views. However, another patient may say 'Yes it puzzles me as well. Sometimes, I think that it could be serious'. You can then ask 'On those occasions when you think it could be serious what exactly do you think about'. She may reply 'I keep thinking it must be cancer'. You should next ask if she would like to discuss her fears that it could be cancer. This will help her develop and enlarge her awareness. Challenging inconsistencies in the history may fail to dent denial. It is then useful to ask the patient 'Have you at any point, even for a split second, considered that your illness may be more serious than you so far believed'? You can then try to develop her awareness.

Doctor: You have told me that all is going well with you and that there are no problems.

But can I ask you, is there ever a moment, even for a fraction of time, when you considered that things may not work out so well?

Patient: Yes, I suppose there is.

Doctor: When is that?

Patient: In the early hours of the morning.

Doctor: Would you mind telling me about that?

Patient: Sometimes, just as I am trying to get off to sleep I panic that I may have Aids.

Doctor: Could you bear to tell me about your panics?

Patient: Most of the time I tell myself that the sweats, tiredness and swollen glands are due to glandular fever. But when I am lying there I have this terrible dread that it could be due to Aids.

Doctor: Are there any other reasons why you think it could be Aids rather than glandular fever?

Patient: When I was overseas on a business trip I had an affair. I didn't take precautions. I worry that I could have contracted Aids then.

Doctor: Your worry that you might have Aids seems to be upsetting to you.

Patient: It is. That's why I have been trying to put it to the back of my mind. But the more these symptoms continue the more I think it's a strong possibility.

This patient has indicated that he has considered that his symptoms are due to a more serious cause than glandular fever. By asking if he has ever had any doubts he is able to articulate this and develop his awareness.

DEALING WITH ANGER

When a patient or relative becomes very angry with you you should try to avoid being defensive however tired or fragile you feel.

Doctor: Why have you asked me to see you so urgently?

Relative: Because I am furious.

Doctor: Why are you furious?

Relative: You said you would get him better within four to six weeks. He's been here three months now and he is getting worse. I am beginning to think that he is not going to get better.

Doctor: That's not fair. We've been doing our best, I can't help it if things don't turn out as I expected.

Relative: But you are supposed to be the expert, you're the one who suggested he would be better within a few weeks.

Doctor: Yes I did but . . .

Relative: You really shouldn't mislead people. You call yourself an expert. You clearly don't know what you're talking about.

The doctor was defensive because he had tried his best to help the patient and felt the relative was being unfair to him. Instead of being defensive try to stay calm and begin by acknowledging the anger that the relative or patient is displaying. You should then seek to establish the intensity of the patient's or relative's anger before exploring all the contributory reasons. Make sure you have elicited all the reasons before you seek to resolve any of them.

Doctor: You seem angry at the moment.
Relative: You're right I'm livid.
Doctor: Just how livid have you been?
Relative: I have never been so livid, I can't find words to express how angry I am, I could scream and scream and scream.
Doctor: What is it that's been making you feel so angry?
Relative: We only brought our mother here because we heard that you knew what you were doing. We were confident that she wouldn't die in pain especially as one of your nurses promised us that. She's been here two weeks but she is in even greater pain. Nothing you are doing seems to be helping her.
Doctor: I'll try and respond to that complaint but are there any other reasons why you are so angry with us apart from our failure to control her pain?
Relative: Yes, we all think she has been neglected since coming here.
Doctor: In what way?
Relative: When we visit, the nurses seem to be spending a lot of time with other patients and very little with our mother.
Doctor: Are there any other reasons for your anger?
Relative: Are they not enough?
Doctor: Yes, but I just want to check to make sure I have understood all the reasons why you are feeling so angry before I try to respond.

The doctor knows that the patient's relatives were promised effective pain control and so he judges the anger to be rational and justified. He responds as follows:

Doctor: Yes, I'm afraid you are right. Contrary to what we hoped we have failed to control her pain so far and she has been suffering terribly. I am extremely sorry about that but we are continuing to do our best to try and sort it out.
Relative: Your best!
Doctor: Yes, because we are still concerned to try and help her with the pain. I appreciate it must be awful for you to see her suffering like this.
Relative: Awful! What do you know about it?
Doctor: Well, tell me how you see it.
Relative: She's in absolute agony, she can hardly move, she says it's a nightmare and she would be better off dead.
Doctor: I can appreciate why you are so concerned about her. I will certainly review with the team what we are doing with her and try and see if there is any way we can ease her suffering. I will call in a second opinion if we can't improve her situation. I am just sorry we haven't been able to be more effective to this date.
Relative: What about the nurses neglecting her?
Doctor: I'm puzzled about that because our nurses don't normally neglect people. But in view of what you say I'll look into it. I would then like to discuss my findings with you.

Could we meet up again in a few days time?

Relative: Yes, I want it sorting out.

Doctor: In the meantime I'll see what we can do to improve the control of her suffering.

Relative: Thank you.

Despite being faced with a very angry relative the doctor has succeeded in defusing her anger because he has taken her concerns seriously and acknowledged that he would take appropriate action. In other situations the use of these strategies may fail to diffuse the anger. You should then consider whether some of the anger belongs elsewhere.

Doctor: In view of what you said about her suffering, I can accept that you are angry with us for not controlling her pain and neglecting her. But I am concerned that you still seem very angry. I am worried that some of your anger towards me may belong elsewhere, to another situation or another person, could that be possible?

Relative: I keep thinking that this is senseless. Why on earth does she have to suffer in this way. What has she done to deserve it? What kind of a world is it that allows a woman as good as her to have cancer. I suppose when it gets down to it, I am furious that she has cancer and that it has to be an incurable sort.

Doctor: I agree. It seems senseless. No wonder you're angry at her suffering.

Sometimes the irrational element of the anger stems from previous experiences. Consequently enquiry about where the anger might be coming from can have a different outcome.

Doctor: As you are talking to me I get the feeling that some of your anger is more than can be explained by what we have done so far. Could there be anything else that has made you or is making you angry at the moment?

Relative: Yes, there is. I don't think she would have ever ended up here if her doctor had diagnosed it sooner.

Doctor: What do you mean?

Relative: When she was first presented with a lump in the breast she was told it was benign. She went back several times because she still had the lump. Her doctor insisted it was benign. It was only later that the surgeon admitted that it must have been malignant even then and that she would not have had a recurrence of her disease so soon. I keep thinking that she would have lived so much longer if that doctor had diagnosed the cancer sooner. That makes me full of rage and despair.

Doctor: I can understand that but could some of your rage be due to the fact that you lost your daughter?

Relative: Yes, it is. It is so unfair to lose her before she is even thirty.

HANDLING DISTRESS

As you talk to a patient she may become extremely distressed. You should acknowledge this by saying 'I can see you have become very distressed' and invite her to discuss the reasons ('Could you bear to tell me why you are so distressed'?) As she talks about her distress it is important to observe if she can contain it and talk through it or is becoming disorganized by it. If there is any hint that she is being disorganized by it ask 'This seems to be getting too painful for you, can you bear to continue'? She will either indicate 'Yes, it is painful but I would like to continue' or say 'No, it's far too painful, I would rather stop here'. If she indicates it is too painful you should respect this. If she is willing to talk further explore just how distressed she is and the reasons. In exploring her distress use active rather than passive techniques. Otherwise she will remain very distressed.

Here, the doctor uses passive techniques:

Doctor: You say you felt devastated when you lost a breast.
Patient: Yes, devastated.
Doctor: Devastated?
Patient: As devastated as it is possible to be.
Doctor: 'Possible to be'?
Patient: .... (*Silent*)

The patient was put in touch with her feelings of devastation about losing a breast but given no way of rescuing herself from them.

In the following example the doctor uses more active techniques, which allows the woman to talk about the devastation and extricate herself.

Doctor: So you say you feel devastated about losing your breast.
Patient: I am absolutely devastated.
Doctor: What exactly is it about losing a breast that makes you feel devastated? (explore reasons)
Patient: I feel I will never be attractive to a man again. I feel so unfeminine. I can't stand looking at myself in the mirror.
Doctor: Are there any other aspects about losing a breast that make you feel so devastated?
Patient: I feel so vulnerable. I feel that, now that a part of me has been taken away, I am no longer in control of my life.
Doctor: No wonder you feel devastated. Are there any other factors contributing to these feelings?
Patient: No.

Here the patient has been encouraged to define the components that are contributing to her feeling devastated. She then feels better because she feels understood even though no attempt has yet been offered to resolve her concerns. In this way what appears to be overwhelming distress can be reduced to more manageable proportions.

CONCLUSION

These are guidelines to help you deal with difficult communication situations. You need to test them out 'at the sharp end'. The easiest way to validate them is to see what happens to your patients and relatives when you use them. You can also ask the patient or relative at the end of the session 'How do you now feel about things'? By use of these strategies and inviting validation you should be able to get positive feedback that they work and this should encourage you to integrate them within your normal practice. You can also use a small tape recorder to record your sessions and check out your strategies. Such attempts to monitor and improve communication are welcomed by most patients.

SUGGESTED FURTHER READING

Maguire, P. (1985) 'Barriers tó psychological care of the dying', *British Medical Journal* 291: 1711–13.

Maguire, P. and Faulkner, A. (1988) 'Improve the counselling skills of doctors and nurses in cancer care', *British Medical Journal* 297: 847–9.

Rosser, J.E. and Maguire, P. (1982) 'Dilemmas in general practice: the care of the cancer patient', *Social Science and Medicine* 16: 315.

Chapter 7

Communication in terminal illness and bereavement

Averil Stedeford

Twelve years' experience of working with cancer patients and their families has convinced me that they suffer more often from problems in communication about the illness than from any other cause except unrelieved pain. Patients who are very anxious or depressed are often preoccupied with questions about their diagnosis and prognosis, and with how to talk to their relatives and others about these things. Addressing such issues appropriately relieves the psychological distress far more effectively than medication can, but requires more skill from the doctor. Why do we as a profession sometimes manage this aspect of consultation so badly?

When we are with a patient who is suffering intensely from his condition, we can usually retain a measure of detachment by using the defence of saying to ourselves, 'This is not very likely to happen to me, or to someone in my family'. But when we are with someone who is dying or bereaved, this defence is not available to us. We tend to identify with them, and our anxiety level rises. If we recognize this we can compensate for it. If we ignore our anxiety or it remains unconscious, it can result in avoidance behaviours such as buck-passing, not allowing the patient to talk freely, undue abruptness, assuming that the patient does not want to know, inappropriate reassurance or even lying.

A general practitioner knew from a neurologist's report that a young patient of his almost certainly had motor-neurone disease. The young man did not come to the surgery and the doctor did not seek him out. A few months later he happened to see the patient's wife in his partner's antenatal clinic. The couple already had two children and the GP suddenly realized that they might not have embarked on a third pregnancy if they had known the likely diagnosis. When he went to see them he found to his dismay that the husband was much worse but had not consulted because he thought nothing could be done for him. Neither of them had guessed the serious import of his symptoms. When they were told, the wife felt she could not cope with another baby and a husband with a progressive illness, and the couple asked for the pregnancy to be terminated. Both were very resentful that such important information had been withheld from them and that they had to go through the additional trauma of an abortion.

Some mistakes in communication are due to thoughtlessness. One patient, whose bed was next to a sister's desk, learned his diagnosis by overhearing the doctor talking about him on the telephone. Another did so when a new doctor came to talk to him about treatment and he saw that his name-badge indicated that he was from the Department of Radiotherapy. Neither of these patients felt able to reveal what they had learned at once, and they suffered unnecessary anxiety as a result.

Another group of problems is the result of poor organization and liaison between different teams caring for the same person. The general practitioner can set the tone in his referral letter. If the possibility that the condition may be malignant has been discussed and the patient has indicated that he wants to be kept fully informed, letting the hospital doctor know this is very helpful, both to him and the patient. Discharge letters about seriously ill patients should include information about what they have been told and their response. The fact that their doctor knows this makes them feel well cared for, and the GP is more confident in his handling of the follow-up visit. For all this to happen, the notes from which the discharge letter is compiled must be adequate. Similarly, good communication between nurses and social workers in the hospital and those in the community makes for better care. Even within the same ward, a nurse may not know what the doctor has told her patient, or vice versa. A special 'communication sheet' in the notes can be very helpful if it is well used. The death of a patient in hospital should be reported to the GP promptly. Otherwise he may meet a newly bereaved relative and enquire how the patient is getting on.

Much of the difficulty in communication in terminal illness centres around the diagnosis and prognosis. Throughout most of our adult lives, we know more about our personal situation than anyone else does, and we endeavour to control the flow of information about ourselves, deciding what can be known by others and what should remain secret. When a patient consults a doctor and the ensuing investigations show that he has a serious illness, perhaps one from which he will die, the position is different. The new information is about the patient, but it is the doctor who has the control. How they proceed is determined by their assumptions about the contract between them.

THE DOCTOR–PATIENT CONTRACT

There are at least two views about the nature of this contract. Some see it in a technical light, as a transaction between a customer and an expert. Here the patient presents himself to the doctor rather as he presents his car at a garage when he suspects that it is developing a fault. He expects thorough investigation, good treatment, and also full information about the nature of the problem and what is to be done about it. On this basis the doctor knows what to tell, and need only ask himself how he is going to give the information, and when: whether he should give it all at once or in stages.

Others see the doctor more as a parental figure. Here the expectation is that the doctor will take the best possible care of the patient and includes an assumption that he will care for the patient's emotional well-being by handling the information he has about him in the way that will be most beneficial to him in the long run. Both are contracts about trust: on the one hand, trust that the doctor will tell the whole truth; and, on the other, that he will care for the whole person. Sometimes these two will match exactly, the whole truth being the best possible thing for that patient to hear. Often they will not match so neatly and then the physician has to decide what to do. If he decides in an independent or arbitrary way how much it is good for his patient to know, he is not respecting the patient's right to knowledge about himself. The dilemma is that until the patient knows what the information is and feels its impact on him, he cannot be certain whether he would have wanted to be told or not. Therefore the decision-making about the flow of information has to be carried out as a delicate negotiation between doctor and patient in which the doctor tries to ascertain how much the patient wants to know and then makes his disclosures appropriately. Occasionally patients do make it clear beforehand how they think they will want information handled should they become seriously ill. They say things like, 'Don't beat about the bush with me, Doctor. Call a spade a spade'. A few others make it equally clear that they do not want to be told much about their illness, or share in decisions about treatment: 'I'm in your hands, Doctor, I'd rather leave it all to you', they say. But usually the doctor is not lucky enough to have this information beforehand and he must feel his way. Sometimes this can be done in a fairly direct fashion by saying something like: 'I have just got the results of your tests back. Would you like us to talk about them in detail now or shall I just tell you what I think the best treatment will be for your condition?' A question put like this allows the patient to control the information coming to him and also tells him that the physician is willing to talk about the nature of the condition when the patient is ready.

TALKING ABOUT DIAGNOSIS

In the early stages of any serious disease, particularly if a cure is likely, there seems little justification for revealing the diagnosis when the patient has been given ample opportunity to ask and has not done so. When malignant disease does recur after treatment which was aimed at cure, the patient may reproach the doctor for not volunteering the whole truth at the outset, but he is equally likely to be grateful for having been spared months or years of anxiety.

It is seldom appropriate, in my opinion, to tell a patient he has been cured, for example of cancer, if the physician knows it is unlikely to be true. Trust between patient and physician is an essential component in the good doctor–patient relationship. Patients need to know that the doctor understands their condition and is not unduly surprised by new developments. The patient who thinks he has been cured concludes, when he has a recurrence, that his physician did not appreciate the seriousness of his disease, and he then doubts his competence to continue care. There is a temptation to end the consultation after surgery for cancer with a comment like, 'You will be fine now', but gratuitous reassurance can be as inappropriate as gratuitous information. Either may occasionally be given for the sake of the doctor rather than the patient, because he is finding it hard to bear within himself the pain of his knowledge of the poor prognosis. Unrealistic reassurance can be effective in the short term, but later the patient will feel he has been deceived should the optimistic forecast prove to be untrue. If symptoms return, the doctor who can say 'I did know that might happen', and go on to explain what he can now do to help, convinces the patient that his condition has been understood and further development anticipated. Eventually he comes to recognize that his doctor cannot prevent him from dying. At times he will be angry and disappointed with him for this, but if the doctor–patient relationship can survive this phase, he will be upheld by the knowledge that his doctor knows how to minimize his suffering and will care for him right to the end.

THE PATIENT WHO SEEMS NOT TO WANT TO KNOW

As a general rule, it is right to let the patient control the flow of information and to assume that if he does not make use of good opportunities to ask questions, he should not be confronted with the seriousness of his condition. But there are a number of situations where this policy would not be in the patient's best interests. Sometimes the patient does not ask about his prognosis because the possibility of serious illness and death just has not occurred to him; this is particularly true of the patient who is young and fit but who nevertheless has a condition which is going to be rapidly progressive, for instance malignant melanoma which is showing no response to treatment. If he is not told until he is very ill, he is likely to regret that he did not have enough notice to enable him to plan ahead and do some essential things while he was still reasonably well.

Sometimes it is necessary to impress upon the patient that his illness is serious, even life-threatening, so that he can understand why the doctor is recommending treatment which may make him feel worse or have undesirable and permanent side-effects such as sterility or loss of hair.

> Sheila was in her late twenties and had an emergency caesarean section about two weeks before her baby was due. At operation she was found to have cancer of the ovary which had spread widely within her abdomen. Toward the end of her pregnancy she had noticed that she was bigger than with her previous baby, and got rather more tired, but she took little notice of this. The day after operation the gynaecologist told her husband of his findings and their serious significance, but they agreed to give her a little time to recover and enjoy the baby without fear before the news was broken to her. Later I asked her how she reacted: 'I was very upset and very angry that such a thing should happen to me', she said, but she emphasized that it had been essential for her to know the diagnosis: 'I was longing to be at home with the baby, and my little girl. I wanted us as a family to be together again as quickly as possible. Several weeks in hospital seemed crazy to me, especially since I felt perfectly well. If I had not known what was involved, I would certainly have refused treatment.' After she did get home, she found it very hard to come back when further radiotherapy was indicated. She told me how her family almost forced her to agree: 'You'll be dead if you don't', they said. Sheila completed her treatment and was very well when I last heard of her two years later.

Another group of patients who benefit from being told their diagnosis is composed of those who are coping unsuccessfully with the recognition of their serious prognosis while using the defence of denial. The purpose of psychological defences is the reduction of suffering, especially anxiety. If the denying patient is living as well as the limitations of his disease will allow, the defence is serving its purpose and should probably be left alone. But if the patient is saying 'There is nothing wrong with me, doctor', and at the same time exhibiting all the signs of an anxiety state, the defence is ineffective and only causes extra problems.

Nora, a middle-aged woman who had breast cancer, became gradually more ill but steadfastly maintained that there was nothing seriously wrong with her and that she would soon be well. Yet she always looked worried, was unable to settle to anything and had recurrent nightmares of being trapped in a box. She awoke from these feelings when she was desperately trying to push up the lid and escape. All of us felt that she would be less anxious if she could admit that she knew she was going to die, and could talk to us about her fears. Yet she blocked every attempt we made to help her to talk. One day I tried to get round it by asking her opinion about the management of illness in general: 'Do you think it is ever right to tell a patient their diagnosis if they are seriously ill?' I asked. 'Oh no,' she said, 'if you did, it would make them worried and they might have nightmares.' Even then she could not make the link which would enable her to talk about herself, but eventually she did. Another patient, whom she had got to know quite well, died very peacefully. Nora began to talk about this and we used the opportunity to help her to admit that she too had cancer and would one day die. As soon as this could be said, she was able to ask questions about how it would happen, whether it would be painful and how much longer she had. Following this she became almost contented, and active in a more constructive way: knitting and helping her husband at home during the time when she was well enough to be there. The appalling nightmares ceased and did not return during the remaining six months of her life.

CHANGES IN AWARENESS

Nora's story leads naturally to a discussion on the changes in awareness that take place as illness progresses. Even the matter-of-fact person who asks a lot of questions and seems to take in all the answers, seldom accepts the full implication of his diagnosis and prognosis all at once. If it were possible to contemplate simultaneously all the losses that a dying person faces, the result would surely be overwhelming. So it is not surprising that most people cope a step at a time. Even this is not an orderly progression. At times of exacerbation of disease, patients face the prospect of death anew, and make further adjustments. If there is a period when they feel better, they behave and talk as if they may recover after all.

This variability in awareness can be perplexing to professional and family alike. For some patients it signifies that they are not yet ready to face the truth. Thus a discharge letter about Mrs X may tell the GP that she has been fully informed about her diagnosis and prognosis, yet when he visits her she may say, 'Nobody in the hospital would tell me what was wrong with me'. Further questioning may reveal that she remembers part of what she was told but has not grasped its significance. Alternatively, she may deny having been told anything, and her indignation may be taken as an indication that she does want information. If the GP responds by explaining it all again, he may be surprised to hear from his practice nurse a few days later that Mrs X is complaining that no one has talked to her about her illness. Such patients do not want truth, they want reassurance. They will ask around until they get an answer which is more acceptable to them, and they will cling to that. Experience has taught me to counter the comment 'Nobody has told me . . .' with a question like, 'How do you think you are getting on?' If the patient replies that he thinks he is getting worse, I ask him what has happened lately to make him think so. He can be gently led on to reveal that he has seen the signs for himself and drawn his own conclusions. I do not tell him; rather I confirm his opinion if it is correct, or refute it and explain if it is not. Thus the realization comes at his pace.

If the same patient responds to my question with 'I am getting better, aren't I?', I suspect that he is not ready for the truth. In order to reassure him without lying, I try to pick out any aspect of his condition which has improved, and emphasize that. 'Well, it's certainly true that your pain is much better than it was when you first came in' might be a suitable response. If he partly wants to know, he will be sensitive to what was left unsaid, and may ask more. 'But why am I losing so much weight, doctor?' If he wants to maintain his denial, he is likely to tell his family, 'The doctor agreed my pain is improving, so I must be getting better.' When he is ready, he will ask more, and take it in.

Other patients realize the full importance of the seriousness of their condition at a practical and intellectual level at the beginning. They tell those who must be told, and make necessary financial and other arrangements. Then they may surprise everyone by talking and behaving as if they will recover, perhaps planning a holiday abroad. They are using the defence of denial in a constructive way, and they are not unduly anxious.

TALKING ABOUT PROGNOSIS

Almost invariably, the patient who knows that he has a terminal illness asks how much longer he can expect to live. Because uncertainty is so painful and because practical decisions have to be made, pressure is often put upon the physician to offer a firm prognosis. Yet we know that it is very seldom possible to give an accurate forecast. Patients have more faith in the doctor's word in this area than is justified, probably because they feel more secure if they have a definite time limit within which to plan. Relatives may make a great effort if they know it will be for a short time; they may be more sparing in their commitment if they have little idea of what will be involved. Sometimes they almost insist on being given a date. I respond to this by telling them that I honestly do not know and asking them how they would feel if I made a guess. 'Supposing I said it would probably be six months', I say, 'I can imagine you going home and getting out the calendar; counting up the weeks and marking the date when the time is up. How will everyone feel as that day approaches?' As soon as they imagine themselves in that position, they withdraw their request for a date, for most people know of someone who has outlived a prognosis by a matter of years.

Even when the doctor takes particular care to be guarded, the patient tends to select what he hears according to his needs and expectations. A statement like 'You will probably have six months to a year' will be interpreted by the pessimist as 'I have only got six months', whereas the optimist may say to his family 'The doctor said I might live for years'. Patients often need to be told quite firmly that we are unable to make a useful prediction. We should offer them continuing support as they cope with uncertainty.

> Jenny was 36 when a diagnosis of lung cancer was made. She owned a little hair-dressing business, and the income from this contributed to the mortgage she and Cyril had on a rather nice new home. When she had to sell the business, they needed to know what her prognosis was. They did not want the proceeds from the sale of the business to be swallowed up in mortgage repayments, which it would be if Jenny lived for long. There was the education of the two children to think about too. So should they sell the house and buy a smaller one? But if Jenny might only live a few months was it fair to impose on her the added strain of moving? They decided to gamble on the proba-bility that Jenny would die before the money ran out, and that her life insurance would then cope. Money did get tight, especially as Cyril took time off work to nurse her towards the end. The couple appreciated the support their general practitioner gave them through the anxiety that this uncertainty engendered. It did work out, but only just.

UNSATISFACTORY COMMUNICATION AND ITS RESULTS

Among 41 couples I interviewed for research purposes, 8 patients and 10 spouses were dissa-tisfied with the quality of communication with their general practitioner; 13 patients and 11 spouses were dissatisfied about communication with hospital doctors. Only one patient complained of being told more than he wanted to know, and he was a person who needed to maintain denial to cope with his anxiety. All the rest spoke of difficulty in obtaining informa-tion, sometimes after quite persistent attempts. Others said their complaints were not taken seriously enough. The last is a complex issue: two of these patients had carcinoma of the pancreas, which is notoriously difficult to diagnose, and three others were hypochondriacal patients with long histories, where the presenting symptom of cancer was not recognized in the plethora of other complaints. Their resentment was exacerbated, of course, by their belief that if the diagnosis had been made sooner, curative treatment might have been possible.

A few patients who complain that their doctor has not given them enough information, have not actually asked direct questions. 'If he thought I ought to know, he would have told me', one lady said. Others thought that the doctor was 'too busy' and one even said 'He was a nice doctor, but young, and he might have been upset to have to tell me a thing like that' (she had cancer). In some cases the doctor could have made it easier for the patient to ask; in others, the responsibility for the lack of information lay mainly with the patient.

To whom do patients turn when they have made a determined effort to get information from their doctors and have failed? McIntosh in his book *Communication and Awareness in a Cancer Ward* (1977) describes vividly how they learn from each other. They compare notes about investigations, symptoms, and treatment, and draw their own (sometimes quite wrong) conclu-sions. They also use non-verbal clues: how long the doctor spends with them, whether the 'round' passes them by or greets them perfunctorily, the expression on the faces of the staff, the attitudes of their relatives. 'I knew it must be serious because everyone started being so nice to me', said one man.

ASKING OTHER PROFESSIONALS

Rather than resort to guessing games and subterfuges, many patients turn to other members of staff for information when their doctor has failed to answer their questions. Some of them do so by choice. Intimidated by the consultant's manner or the size of his retinue, they feel more comfortable asking the junior doctor who examines them, the technician who takes their blood, the nurse who is making the bed, or the social worker who may have been asked to come and talk about financial matters. Both in general practice and in hospital, this asking of others can be very satisfactory, provided the staff work together as a team with a common policy. Usually patients choose to ask a particular person because they feel more at ease with them than with anyone else. It is our policy that, whoever the member of staff happens to be, he or she should answer the question promptly and as fully as seems right for them, provided they are certain of their facts and they feel reasonably sure they can handle the situation. Afterwards they should report what has transpired to medical and nursing colleagues so that others also know and can follow up the conversation if necessary. If the member of staff feels inadequately equipped to answer the question, he or she should without delay find some one who can. 'I am afraid I can't tell you; you will have to ask the doctor' has sinister implications for the patient. He may have thought for several days before he dared to ask anyone at all, and he should not be kept anxiously waiting for too long.

In the course of the ordinary day's work there arise opportunities for junior staff to learn more about talking with patients. If they can sometimes 'sit in' with seniors when this is being done, or if they can discuss their own interactions with patients with their peers and seniors, perhaps in a group setting, their own skills quickly improve, and mutual trust within the team grows. Many patients value the opportunity to talk about their illness in some detail with staff other than doctors and, provided communication within the team is good, the quality of care improves considerably. So, incidentally, does the sense of job satisfaction felt by the staff.

Problems arise when communication is poor and when policy is unclear or is authoritative but divisive. Junior staff experience considerable stress when a patient asks direct questions and the consultant has decided that the truth must be concealed from him. If the nurse or houseman tells without permission, and is later found out, a reprimand or worse may occur. But in many settings it takes courage for a junior nurse or houseman to challenge authority and say 'Mrs X has asked me her diagnosis today and I think she would be better off if she were told'. Nevertheless, this is a more constructive way of dealing with the situation. Discussion with the consultant or ward sister may reveal that there was other information about the patient's background or personality which was not available to junior staff and which was influencing the decision. Alternatively, the consultant who is acting through prejudice or fear may be prepared to think again, and gradually a change of policy may follow.

In the situations described, the patient suffers too. Having asked a question and got no answer, he judges from the evasive response, the quick reassurance, or the embarrassed expression, that he should not have done so, probably because the answer would be too painful for him to bear. So he remains ignorant, but more afraid than before.

When communication about illness goes wrong, it is often claimed that lack of time and poor working conditions are contributory causes. This may be so, but insensitivity, a reluctance on the part of staff themselves to face the issues involved and ignorance are causes too. With training and encouragement, we could do better than this.

TALKING TO RELATIVES

When a patient visits the doctor with a complaint that could be the first symptom of serious illness, both of them make decisions about what to ask and what to tell. Concurrently they decide either actively or by default whether anyone else shall be informed. Bringing a relative or friend and asking that they be included in the consultation should ensure that information is shared from the beginning, but often it does not. Several of the research couples who attended together and asked direct questions reported that they had to press very hard to obtain answers. With more reticent couples, or when the patient attended alone, the doctors were commonly guarded in what they said initially, and found an opportunity to say more to the spouse later. Of the 41 research couples, 9 were told the diagnosis separately. In this small series the measure of satisfaction about communication reported by couples was not influenced by whether or not they were told together.

TELLING RELATIVES MORE THAN THE PATIENT

The practice of telling relatives more than the patient about diagnosis and prognosis is only justified if they ask and the patient, given ample opportunity, does not. When relatives are interviewed separately, they sometimes request or even insist that the patient is not told his diagnosis. This puts the doctor in a difficult position, particularly if he suspects that his patient already wants to know or is likely to ask direct questions in the future. His first duty is to his patient, but it is important to maintain good rapport with the family if at all possible.

There are a number of reasons why relatives ask the doctor not to tell and exploring these patiently may resolve the problem. They may have been advised previously that it is unwise to reveal the truth to patients.

> Daphne, a married woman in her late thirties, had breast cancer. She was told her diagnosis at her explicit request and shared it with her husband. When her mother found out that she knew, she angrily demanded to see a doctor, saying that her daughter would be demoralized by what we had done and that we should have consulted her first. It transpired that two years previously her own husband had died of laryngeal cancer. The surgeon had strongly advised her not to tell her husband his diagnosis and she had kept the secret from him for almost two years, at great cost. She and her daughter were very close, and Daphne did not know whether to side with her mother or with us. The mother was angry with us, not only because she felt we had done something harmful to her daughter, but also because our policy caused her to question the value of what she had done for her husband.

This incident could have been avoided only if we had seen Daphne's mother as well as her husband, soon after admission. Such extended care is not always possible, but the case provides a salutary reminder that the parents of adult patients sometimes need our consideration as much as husbands or wives, and children.

Relatives may believe that the patient will lose hope and stop fighting if he knows the diagnosis. Enquiring about how he has coped with any previous crises may reveal background information useful in influencing how his questions should be answered if and when he does ask. A history of previous depressive illness is not a contraindication to telling the truth; I have known some such patients cope very well. One said to me 'This is much easier than depression. Everyone knows what I have got, and they help me. When I was depressed, nobody understood'. Some patients do go through a crisis of hopelessness soon after they are told, but most emerge from this in a short time and some come out with a determination to fight which is made all the stronger by their knowledge of the odds.

Often relatives do not want the patient to be told because they know intuitively that while he remains in ignorance they can defend themselves against their own grief by keeping up a cheerful facade. They justify this to themselves by saying that they are doing it for the sake of the patient. In fact they are afraid that sharing the knowledge might be unbearably painful for them. Quite often the patient has guessed and he too is pretending, for the sake of the family, and therefore denying himself the opportunity of asking all the questions his secret knowledge has raised in his mind.

Relatives sometimes insist that a patient does not know the truth when there are many indications to staff that he does. I have found it useful to point out to them that he seems to me to be the sort of person who has probably thought a lot about the course of his illness, put two and two together, and drawn his own conclusions. When they consider this idea they often remember little clues he has given them which they ignored before. He may have tested the family by making remarks like 'Don't assume I'll be here forever!' in a way that could either be taken seriously or dismissed as a joke. Recalling something of this kind makes relatives begin to recognize that he might already know. Often they then agree that the doctor may tactfully explore how much the patient has guessed, and answer truthfully any questions that follow. They need to be reassured that he will only go as far as the patient wants and not take a blunt or confronting approach. They also appreciate it if he promises to inform them of the outcome of the interview. If they are left in ignorance, they are apprehensive each time they visit, wondering whether they should maintain their facade or prepare themselves for a very different sort of conversation.

Sometimes doctors advise against telling when relatives would rather be open. This causes problems of a different kind.

Marion was 39 and had a brain tumour. Her symptoms progressed rapidly and she was taken unconscious to theatre for emergency surgery within 48 hours of the beginning of her illness. The neurosurgeon could only partially excise the tumour and he told David, her husband, about her poor prognosis. Without any discussion the neurosurgeon stated that he had decided that she should be told only that she had a cyst and that radiotherapy would cure it. Marion and David had shared everything important up to then, and David really wanted her to know as much about her condition as he did. He felt that they had faced things together in the past and would be able to do so again. But he had been so shocked by the disastrous events that had overtaken them so unexpectedly that he did not think clearly when the surgeon spoke to him, and he felt unable to object. She was very glad to hear that she would soon be much better, and although David still wanted to tell her the truth, he was reluctant to spoil her pleasure in the first good weeks.

Initially she did do well, but soon she stopped improving and began to wonder why her efforts in physiotherapy no longer produced results. When she began to deteriorate, she thought she was not trying hard enough and became depressed, and sometimes suicidal. By then her personality had changed somewhat and David felt she no longer had the resources to cope with the truth. When she came in to our care she was frightened, sometimes paranoid and often confused. We could not tell her then because we could not be certain that she was able to concentrate long enough to take in all we said. She might have understood the bad news but been unable to accept the reassurance we could offer about the care and help that was available. We already knew that when she was paranoid we could not comfort her. So we had to agree with David that it was now too late to tell. We managed her distress as well as we could with drugs, but she died frightened and isolated. Because they had been unable to share, David could not support her as he would have liked, and he was full of regret.

When we discussed it afterwards, we recognized that knowing the truth from the beginning might have produced quite a different sequence of events. Initially, Marion would have been as sad as David, but they could have planned their limited future together. She might have been more pleased with the degree of recovery she achieved. She would not have blamed herself when progress ceased, nor made such vigorous and futile efforts to rehabilitate herself. Because she did not realize that she had a disease that could account for her deterioration, she had to find another cause, and she blamed us. Later, knowing intuitively that she was dying, she said in her paranoia 'You are killing me'.

During an initial consultation, especially when patient and partner are seen separately, the doctor may discover that one or both are dissatisfied about communication between them. An offer to see them together may help them to improve this. Others, having talked the matter through with the doctor individually, would prefer to share their knowledge with each other in privacy, and they should be supported in this. Once this has happened, the couple can begin to make plans.

They can settle details about finances and they can ask more freely for help from the extended family. Even delicate questions like 'Do you want burial or cremation?', or 'How would you feel if I married again?', may be asked and answered. A husband or wife who is about to leave his or her partner with many responsibilities, particularly when there are young children, usually feels guilty. Planning how the surviving spouse will cope relieves some of this guilt, and the bereavement is also made a little easier.

Andrew lived for just 11 weeks after the diagnosis of lung cancer was made. Mary, his wife, was a graduate, but was not working as they had a big family. Together they decided that she should return to college for a year to become a fully trained teacher. In this way her career would give her most free time when her children were at home. They worked out a way for her to finance that year, and they prepared the children for what was going to happen. Some months after Andrew's death, Mary told me 'It was knowing that I was doing what we had both planned that kept me going. It was awful, but I almost felt he was behind me, encouraging me. How I would have coped if we hadn't talked like that I just can't imagine'.

When a couple have just faced together the fact that one of them is likely to die, they often choose not to tell anyone else for a little while, until they have regained their equilibrium and adjusted to the situation themselves. But before long they turn their attention to the extended family. 'How shall we prepare the children?' they ask; and 'When shall we break the news to the parents?' Often they turn to the doctor, nurse or social worker for help with this too.

TELLING THE CHILDREN

There are many variables that influence the way children are prepared, or not prepared, for the death of a parent. It would be common sense to assume that the most powerful deciding factor was the age of the child, but evidence from the 19 couples in my study who had children aged under 18 suggests that the most important factors are the parents' own attitude to death and to openness with children in general, and the amount of support they receive from the extended family. One father began to prepare a little boy of 4 for his mother's death a year before it occurred. Another couple did not tell their daughter and son, aged 16 and 20, until a week before their father died.

Families who are open from the beginning seem on the whole to manage better. The case of Jenny and Cyril illustrates this. Jenny said that as soon as they had been told that she had cancer they decided to tell their children.

We decided immediately that we would tell the children. They are 13 and 16. My daughter was about to go on holiday and we thought that it was best to tell her because we did not know quite how long I had to live. She was very worried. It was only fair to give her the choice. In actual fact she didn't want to go.

I asked her how they took the news.

Well obviously, my husband had to tell them. They were extremely upset of course. They had one day off school each with Cyril, then after that it has been marvellous. They seem to accept it and we talk about it quite openly. I think it is by far the best way because you talk it out of your system, and you don't mope about it too much.

Many families are not as open as this. Often they experience conflict between their wish to confide and be close (especially if they are a family that has not had major secrets before) and their desire to protect those they love from distress. They also want to protect themselves from seeing the sadness which their news will inevitably evoke. They rationalize the decision not to tell in a variety of ways, and they may need help to think through the possible repercussions of the course they plan to adopt.

When talking with parents about telling their children, it is important to help them realize that they cannot wholly control what their children will find out. One couple confided in close friends whose own child overheard them discussing the situation. The next day a little girl learned about her daddy's brain tumour in the playground at school, and her parents then realized how much better it would have been if they could have told her themselves.

Often children realize something is seriously wrong but also sense that their parents do not want them to know. In their ignorance they may even imagine the situation is worse than it really is. If they guess the truth they may confide in other children, or a teacher, and may succeed in concealing their anxiety at home. This enables the parents to deny that the children know, and such parents may be quite angry with the doctor who suggests otherwise. More often such children keep their fears to themselves, and their anxiety may reveal itself in physical symptoms or deterioration in school work. Asking about the children should be part of the care of a parent who is seriously ill. This may lead to a request for help in preparing them. It is not often appropriate to give advice but rather to work out with the parents what they would like to say and how they would cope with the likely consequences. They appreciate hearing about how other families have coped in similar circumstances. Sometimes it is right to offer a family session. However, many parents gain courage from talking the matter through with a professional helper and then feel able to break the news to the children at home when a suitable occasion arises rather than have it happen at a meeting with a stranger. They appreciate knowing that they can come back for continuing support, and they often report a certain pride in their unexpected ability to manage something that seemed so daunting before.

Adolescents do appreciate talking to the doctor alone, and they often reveal a much deeper understanding of their parents than most would give them credit for. Some whom I met had already asked themselves how much they should try to take the place of the dying parent, supporting the surviving mother or father or caring for younger siblings. They have to weigh this against their increasing need for independence and continuing education. Sometimes their sudden 'maturity' is a defence against grief which they would regard as childish. Promiscuity and delinquency are more extreme responses to the threat of losing a parent, or to bereavement.

If the well parent is too preoccupied in attending to the needs of the dying spouse, the children may feel doubly abandoned. The help of relatives, especially grandparents, is very valuable here, and the knowledge that they are useful assuages their own grief a little. Where there are no family members to support the children, a social worker or health visitor may help to fulfil this role for a time, until the parent is again able to give enough. Church-going families are often helped by clergy, youth club leaders, etc., and some schoolteachers also make a major contribution to a child's welfare during a crisis of this kind. The routine of school can provide an area of stability while home feels insecure. Most parents make a point of informing teachers of the illness, so that due allowance is made if the child's work falls below its usual standard, or he develops other problems. All children suffer when they lose a parent, but if they are well supported and do not have to cope with too many other changes or losses at the same time (such as moving house or changing school), their natural resilience may allow them to emerge from their grief and continue their development satisfactorily.

Older patients with adult children sometimes need help too. Some of these parents are reluctant to confide in their offspring, protecting them as if they had never grown up. Others find it hard to accept the role reversal implicit in receiving care from their children. They regard themselves as a burden, and sometimes deprive their sons and daughters of opportunities to help when they would most willingly have done so. Talking these attitudes over with the parent may help him or her to accept support from the children. If they do not, they may cause them more suffering, not less, and during bereavement they too will say 'If only I had known ...'.

TELLING PARENTS

How soon parents are told about the serious illness of a son or daughter depends not only on the closeness of the relationship but also on whether they are perceived as supportive or dependent. In close families there arises conflict between the wish to confide in parents and the wish to protect them from suffering, especially if they are elderly or ill. Where the parent has already had, for instance, a heart attack, and is therefore perceived as particularly vulnerable, patients say things like 'I just couldn't tell him, it might kill him.' Sharing painful information makes it seem more real and inescapable, and the apparently genuine wish to protect parents may represent a rationalization of reluctance to face the truth or to see the parents upset. However, parents who are kept in ignorance until their child is dying or dead suffer far more shock and are also deprived of opportunities to offer help or comfort and to say goodbye. Most patients, when asked to consider this point of view, decide to tell.

> Jenny and Cyril, who prepared their children so well, were anxious about Cyril's mother, whose husband had died two years previously, after which she had moved to be near them. She had arthritis and depended on them for transport and for most of her social contacts. When Jenny became ill, Cyril wanted to devote most of his attention to her and at first felt guilty about doing less for his mother. However, she was very understanding and actually discovered that she could do more for herself than she thought. A neighbour who was asked to help became a friend and introduced her to other women of the same age, so she became more part of the community. The elderly are very grieved at losing a child, sensing that the natural order of events has been reversed, and often they feel guilty at remaining alive. Cyril's mother's new friends of her own generation supported her through this experience, and enabled her to be of more help emotionally to him and his children.

Where relationships are strained, the situation is different. A daughter who perceives her mother as over-protective or possessive may delay telling her for as long as possible, fearing that she will insist on coming to 'help' and will take over the household, handle the children in a different way, or alienate the husband and divide the couple. In poor marriages, and also in very young couples where the bond with the parents is stronger than the new relationship, patients sometimes turn to parents for support, leaving the spouse feeling rejected and jealous. Among my patients, a husband who was afraid this might happen dissuaded his wife from confiding by telling her that it would be cruel to distress her parents with such news.

In divided families, doctors, social workers and others can inadvertently get caught up in rivalries and subterfuge. When relatives ask for an interview, it is wise to check with the patient first. He may wish to retain control of the spread of news through his family and to prevent relatives who are not on speaking terms from suddenly finding themselves one on each side of his bed!

BEREAVEMENT

So far in this chapter the focus has been on the dying patient and his family. Once death has occurred, the family has a new set of needs. Even those who have been expecting it for a long time often find the reality of death shocking when it occurs. If they have been present, they may need to spend time at the bedside, letting the reality sink in and saying their last goodbye. Some appreciate the chance to help the nurse to wash and clothe the body, as the last intimate service they can give. When a death takes place in hospital, relatives who have not been present have to be told, and this duty often falls to the nurse or doctor on duty at the time. If the next of kin is likely to be alone when they receive the phone call, it is wise to plan with the family beforehand who should be the one to break the news.

When the relatives arrive at the hospital, they need to be seen in a quiet place. They often want to know details of the last hours, and if the death has come sooner than expected they may need an explanation. If a member of staff unfamiliar to them is on duty when the death occurs, it may be better to break the news briefly and offer them an appointment later with someone with whom they have talked before. Whoever sees them should recognize that they need time to react in their own way and be listened to, before they are given the practical information they must have about the death certificate, how to make funeral arrangements, etc.

Relatives should be offered an opportunity to see the body, and they should be accompanied when they do this, if they so wish. Paying last respects in this way helps to make the death real and makes problems due to delayed grief less likely. Even little children may benefit from the chance to say goodbye to a parent or grandparent, and families should be helped to consider this possibility and supported if they choose to let it happen. Bereaved children, and particularly adolescents, are often angry later if they have been inappropriately protected from being involved in the last illness and death of a loved relative.

Breaking the news of a sudden death in an accident or disaster can never be done in a way that does not cause distress. Anyone to whom this task falls must be prepared for a variety of reactions, many of which are irrational. It is not possible to take in immediately the full meaning of the event. There may be an initial calm when questions are asked, or there may be shock and utter bewilderment. Some will be concerned with a trivial event that cannot now take place, like a child who asked 'Now who will take me to the circus tomorrow?' This does not indicate any lack of love for the deceased, but rather a total incapacity to take in the enormity of what has happened.

There will be an urgent need for more information, and often the person who has brought the news has few details to offer. He is likely to be the target for the anger and frustration that the newly bereaved person feels, and one of his tasks is to tolerate this emotion and help the distressed person to contain it. It is very unpleasant to be accused of something that is not one's fault, but defending oneself in this situation increases the anger. The professional person must recognize that he is dealing with a displacement of powerful emotions onto himself. In the face of disaster everyone would like to undo what has happened, and each has to face his or her helplessness and impotence. In some ways it is easier for those who can be active, doing what *is* possible, than it is for those who can only wait. They need help to express their feelings safely as they emerge, and to contain them when they become unmanageable. Continuing contact with one person who will listen and wait with them, liaise for them with any officials involved and help them to plan the next step contributes to keeping the distress within bounds. A trusted friend or relative can give support of a different kind, and contacting such a person should be encouraged, even though their arrival at the scene may seem initially to add to the confusion.

Immediately after a death the task of the professionals involved is to ensure that the bereaved relatives have the support they need to get through the initial shock and proceed with the practical matters that have to be accomplished. Later a decision has to be made about what after-care, if any, will be required and who should take responsibility for this.

First an assessment must be made of how much the bereaved are at risk of experiencing a traumatic or abnormal grief reaction. This depends on the severity of the loss they have sustained and its meaning for them, and also on what resources they have to draw on, both within themselves and in their family and social network. Bereavement is part of normal life and many people will get through it satisfactorily without professional intervention. It is often right for the general practitioner or another person involved with the family to continue a monitoring function to ensure that this is happening and to intervene if necessary.

Where there is a lack of family or social support, or the risk of a severe grief reaction is judged to be high, follow-up will be needed. Here good liaison is essential between those involved at the time of the death and those who can offer long-term care to relatives. The wishes of the latter and their willingness to accept help must also be taken into account, of course. Terminal care is complete when those caring for the patient who has died have done their best to ensure that the bereaved family will cope as well as possible. They must choose the right level of care from the wide range available and communicate the nature of the needs and problems as accurately as possible. This hand-over is part of grief-work of the professionals too and enables them to move on to the next patient and family who will come into their care.

Much of this chapter has been taken from the author's book: Stedeford A. (1984) *Facing Death: Patients, Families, and Professionals*, London: William Heinemann Medical Books.

SUGGESTED FURTHER READING

McIntosh, J. (1977) *Communication and Awareness in a Cancer Ward*, London: Croom Helm.
Stedeford, A. (1981) 'Couples facing death; II, unsatisfactory communication', *British Medical Journal* 283: 1098–101.
Worden, W.J. (1983) *Grief Counselling and Grief Therapy*, London: Tavistock.

Chapter 8

Crisis intervention with cancer patients

Nira Kfir and Maurice Slevin

For many cancer patients and their families, the diagnosis is a time of great stress, when they are faced by a new situation from which it may seem there is no escape. Most patients for whom a realistic curative option is available may be able to see the light at the end of the tunnel, even if the route is different. Unfortunately, many patients may have to live with the knowledge that they are unlikely to be cured and face the reality of a limited life expectancy, together with often severe effects on their quality of life of both the disease and its treatment.

In many respects the reactions to a diagnosis of cancer are similar to any other life crisis, although there are also differences specific to the cancer situation. If so, the basic principles of crisis intervention should apply to this situation as much as to any other life crisis such as bereavement or divorce.

A MODEL OF CRISIS AND HOW IT APPLIES TO THE CANCER PATIENT

People often use the term 'crisis' as an exaggerated metaphor which does not differentiate it from a stressful time in life. A model of crisis was developed by Kfir after Israel's Yom Kippur war in October 1973, to work with newly bereaved families and see them through the first year of bereavement. It was developed as a practical model within an Adlerian framework. In this model, crisis is characterized by three aspects and only if all these three occur can it be related to as a crisis. These aspects are:

1   Lack of information in a totally new situation.
2   Aloneness and a sense of lack of support.
3   A feeling that there are no options available.

When faced with a diagnosis of cancer the majority of people go through a phase of shock, but this is usually short-lived and resolves spontaneously. Despite this rapid recovery from the initial shock there can be few patients who do not suffer a feeling of a lack of information, support and options and hence feel lost and uncertain. For some this feeling may continue for years.

Lack of information in a totally new situation

When a cancer patient is informed of the diagnosis, the information he receives does not resemble any other learning experience he has had. Faced with this situation, the patient immediately tries to reach for a ready response only to find that there is none. In most stressful situations relating to work, relationships, etc., an automatic response is immediately available. Faced with cancer, however, people press the 'automatic button' and find that they do not have a response to the diagnosis. It is not just the newness or the lack of the ready response, but rather the awareness that the information they have just been given may be critical, progressive and irreversible. This creates a feeling of 'I don't know what to do' which results in anxiety which can evolve into panic.

The first reaction is a sense of a lack of information. One might argue that there is so much information out in the open about cancer that people can hardly claim ignorance. This general information is totally different from personal experience. What patients mean by lack of information is 'I do not know what will happen to me', 'How will I cope?', 'Will I survive this?'. People also have to cope with previous information; such as cancer is always fatal, treatment is intolerable, you are not punished for nothing, people will avoid you, it is disgusting, it smells of death. It is often very difficult for individuals to assimilate their own diagnosis within this frame of reference because it is simply too alarming.

The newly diagnosed patient initially asks 'why? what has caused it? what for?'. Most patients are faced with no clear answers. Having failed to find a physiological reason for the cancer, they often look for psychological or moral ones. 'Why me?' is the most common, routed in moralistic 'reward and punishment' thinking. Again there is usually no answer.

The patient is then faced with the invasion of all sorts of experts into their life. The mystery of cancer makes the experts even more powerful but at the same time more doubtful. People know that in spite of their expertise, even the specialists are often faced with uncertainty and there is no way of being sure about the results of treatment or about life expectancy. Faced with a lack of information, the inability to understand or justify the cancer and the need to place your trust in the hands of experts who themselves can often give no sure answers results in an intense sense of lack of control. Patients receive conflicting messages about what they should do from a wide a variety of sources ranging from their next-door neighbour to the news media. These include:

You have to trust your doctor.
Don't tell anyone you are ill.

Change your life now that you have cancer.
Most people with cancer die sooner or later.

Look for a second opinion.
It is important to talk about your illness to get support.
Go on as if nothing has happened.
They are making progress, many people are now cured.

The lack of control, the progressive anxiety and the lack of reassuring information, together with the need to trust the experts totally, are the first dimensions of the crisis.

Aloneness and a sense of lack of support

No matter how close and supportive the patient's family and friends are, it doesn't take the patient long to realize that 'this is only happening to me' or, as one patient said, 'only one of us is dying'. Complaints of this sort are very hard on the family and sick people may seem ungrateful or inconsiderate of the difficulties and anxieties of their supporters. This sense of loneliness and lack of support is therefore unrelated to the attitude of friends but to the feelings of the patient himself. Often for the first time in their lives, people experience what it means to be truly alone and for most people this is a very frightening realization. Having to face the uncertainty of survival often makes relationships and former roles seem irrelevant.

'No options' – the sense of finality

This third characteristic of any crisis is the feeling that one is running out of solutions and options. In the beginning the only option the patient is looking for is full recovery. Even in those cancers which respond very favourably to treatment, no one can guarantee full recovery or promise that a recurrence will never occur. Although it is often stated that 'cancer is the chronic disease with the highest cure rate', this is not a sufficient solution to the problem of the individual patient. For the patient with a cancer that generally does not respond well to treatment, especially if they are told by the doctor that there is nothing that can be done, it is very easy to feel that there are really no options available and that there is no way out of this situation.

CRISIS INTERVENTION

The principles of crisis intervention in this model are firmly based on helping people in the three areas which characterize the crisis itself and comprise providing information, emotional support and options. It is hypothetical that this model may also be useful in dealing with cancer patients who are not in crisis but who are distressed and anxious.

Information

Despite the wide availability of many general publications about cancer, many patients are ill-informed about their disease. Some wish to remain so, and their wishes should be respected, but many are forced into this position. Nervous, bewildered and upset they may not know the 'right' questions to ask their doctor or have the initiative to seek out information. Patients need to be given a certain amount of general information freely which they can then follow up with further questions or not, as they wish.

Information is a major means of helping people cope with this totally 'new' situation and the feeling of lack of control. Patients' needs for information differ but most need a general explanation of what cancer is, how their cancer affects them and what the current treatments available for cancer comprise. Even if none of the standard treatments, i.e. surgery, radiotherapy or chemotherapy, is relevant to that particular patient, having this information can significantly help at an emotional level in giving them a sense of control over their life. In a similar way, providing people with information about what research is going on into new cancer therapies puts their situation in perspective and allows them to feel a sense of hope that new treatments may become available in time to help them. However unlikely this may be in practice, it is always a real possibility and this information can be very powerful.

The changes that take place in the cancer patient's life are not only those related to the disease and treatment but also to the changes in their relationships. Many patients need information to help them understand why difficulties may arise with their spouses and close friends and to understand the anger and frustration in relationships, love and sex which often arise. To realize that these feelings are experienced by many people and are in many respects a normal human response to illness can be very reassuring and relieve feelings of guilt and depression. People often need information about how to talk to children and older parents as well as dealing with work colleagues, insurance and so on.

Not all information is necessarily helpful. It is the common experience of cancer doctors and borne out by the enquiries to BACUP Cancer Information Service that the majority of patients with cancer do not wish to discuss their own prognosis or to deal with their likely life expectancy. To give a patient a finite time limit is likely not only to be inaccurate but may also devalue and discolour their lives. In giving personal medical information it is very important to maintain hope. Patients respect honesty but this is not incompatible with an emphasis on the more hopeful, even if less likely, aspects of a patient's position.

Emotional support

Emotional support is clearly of tremendous importance for cancer patients. Equally obviously there is a limit to what the health services can provide in this area. Much will depend on the individual's family and friends. Service providers have an informative role, as discussed above, in encouraging patients to make the most of their own resources. Seeking, and accepting, support are not skills in which healthy self-reliant individuals are normally adept or feel comfortable with. These skills can and should be taught to cancer patients and their families.

Emotional support is given to the patient by their knowing that there are people they can turn to who will 'be there' for them. Patients often talk of the emotional support provided by the nurses and doctors simply by knowing they are available at the end of the telephone or when they come to clinic. Specialist cancer units, by providing a large number of staff with a special understanding of what their patients are going through, can provide a flexible, open and accessible system to meet these emotional needs. They are also in a better position to offer patients emotional support services such as counselling or support groups. Many patients, even those not initially attracted to the idea, have derived immense benefit from sharing experiences, hopes and fears with others in a similar position. It is a very different kind of emotional support to that provided by a patient's family and friends who don't have cancer, but no less necessary. Many also benefit from talking through their problems with a well-trained counsellor.

Options

It often seems to a patient with newly diagnosed cancer that there are few or no options. Doctors make a major error if they tell a patient there is absolutely nothing that can be done and also that there is nothing they can do to help themselves. The major option that can be given to patients is to encourage them towards regaining control over their lives. While it is clearly not possible to tell patients that this will result in the disease retreating, it is realistic and honest to encourage people to try and live as healthy a life style as possible on the basis that this can only be good for them. In this light, suggesting to people to eat a generally well-balanced healthy diet, to take regular exercise within the context of what is possible for them and to try to deal with anxiety and feelings of despondency using well-established relaxation techniques, results in their feeling that they can regain a sense of purpose and control over their lives. These options should be provided by conventional doctors and not only in the context of alternative medicine.

Adding 'life to years' is in WHO terms (WHO, 1985) as much a health service priority as adding 'years to life'. It sometimes seems that the giving of advice on healthy lifestyles and self-help is an accepted part of the medical role in every disease except cancer. Possibly the advances in high technology and treatment have increased the emphasis on cure at the expense of simple care. Yet in cancer this advice is much needed. Shattered and depressed by their diagnosis and by continuing treatment and uncertainty, patients need help in regaining a sense of control and well-being. Very aware of how precious life is, they are naturally receptive to ideas about how its quality might be enhanced.

It is often left to alternative medicine to provide the simple options discussed above. Unfortunately they are sometimes very extreme and are usually linked to unproven methods of intervention, much to the bewilderment of a desperate and very vulnerable patient group. But it need not and should not be so. It is possible for cancer doctors to provide patients with realistic ways of doing things for themselves without offering false hope or resorting to pseudo-science.

APPLICATION OF THE MODEL

These principles of crisis intervention can be applied in everyday oncological practice by cancer doctors and nurses provided they have an appreciation of the emotional needs of their patients as well as the time and expertise to deal with them. Providing information, emotional support and options are a simple and practical means of intervention.

ACKNOWLEDGEMENTS

The authors would like to thank Dr Ann Dennison, a patient, for her help with writing this article and Vivienne Griffiths and Fiona Whitehead for preparing the manuscript.

SUGGESTED FURTHER READING

Harris, J. (1985) *The Value of LIfe*, London: Routledge & Kegan Paul.

Kfir, N. (1981) 'Impass-Priority Therapy', in R.J. Corsini (ed.) *Handbook of Innovative Therapies of the Seventies*, New York: John Wiley & Sons.

Plant, H., Richardson, J., Stubbs, L., Lynch, D., Ellwood, J., Slevin, M. and De Haes, H. (1987) 'Evaluation of a support group for cancer patients and their families and friends', *British Journal of Hospital Medicine* 39: 317–20.

Slevin, M.L. (1987) 'Talking about cancer: how much is too much?', *British Journal of Hospital Medicine* 39: 56–9.

Slevin, M.L., Terry, Y., Hallett, N., Jefferies, S., Lauder, S., Plant, R., Wax, H. and McElwain, T. (1988) 'BACUP, the first two years: evaluation of a national cancer information service', *British Medical Journal* 297: 669–72.

Chapter 9

The diagnosis of patients at risk of psychiatric disorder

Russell Blacker

A significant proportion of the general population in Western society are psychiatrically unwell at some point in their lives. Estimates vary according to which diagnostic criteria are used but approximately 1 in 10 persons receive treatment at some point in their lives from a psychiatrist and at least twice as many are treated by their GP. An indication of the quantity and kind of psychiatric morbidity found within the general population is shown by one American Epidemiological Catchment Area Survey in 1984 in which, over a six-month period, more than 15 per cent of the population were found to have experienced a psychiatric disorder. The majority of this morbidity was *affective* in type (6 per cent), a category within which major depressive disorder held the largest share. An additional 5 per cent of the population met diagnostic criteria for alcohol dependence whilst 3 per cent suffered from various neurotic disorders. Only 1 per cent were found to suffer from schizophrenia and related psychoses, whilst 1 per cent were judged to have severe cognitive impairment (dementia).

Previous research has shown that persons with psychiatric conditions are especially likely to consult their general practitioner. There is thus a natural tendency for those with these disorders to concentrate in GPs' surgeries, and surveys usually report a rate for psychiatric disorder amongst GP attenders of 25 to 30 per cent. Similar rates are also obtained in hospital settings. Only a small proportion (probably less than a tenth) of these patients are referred on to psychiatrists and thus it is in the interest of those working in general medical settings to become familiar with the diagnosis and management of the kinds of psychiatric disorders from which their patients are likely to suffer.

Selective referral factors determine what kinds of psychiatric disorder are most commonly encountered in different areas of the medical services. Psychiatrists tend to concentrate on the more severe and flamboyant conditions such as schizophrenia, manic-depressive disorder and severe forms of neurosis. Those working in general medical/surgical hospital settings, on the other hand, will more commonly encounter patients suffering from acute confusional states, alcohol and drug withdrawal, major depressive disorder and deliberate self-harm.

Those in general practice will see proportionally more patients suffering from mild to moderate depression, anxiety and phobic disorders, dementia and personality disorder. The current tendency in medical and nursing training schemes is to expose students selectively to patients found within psychiatric services which may therefore not be particularly useful. This basic training may explain why so many (up to a third or more) of patients with psychiatric disorders in hospital and general medical settings escape detection by their doctors. The obvious solution to this problem would be to revise the training programmes, although research has shown that it is also necessary for clinicians to exercise diagnostic vigilance and to be prepared to interview patients and examine their mental state if the true diagnoses are to be identified.

An additional but important reason for the failure to detect psychiatric disorder is the problem of 'somatization', i.e. the tendency for those with emotional or psychological disorders to present with physical complaints. Since this is a common phenomenon it is important to get to grips with the concept of how patients 'present' and why.

PRESENTATION

A recent study of patients presenting consecutively to five GPs at a north London health centre (n = 2,225) found that 35 per cent of the sample met DSM III criteria for formal psychiatric disorder. Two-thirds of those with psychiatric disorders were presenting with complaints that were purely 'somatic' in type and thus contained no emotional or psychological statements at all. Analysis showed that the patients who presented in this way were more likely to be young or elderly, to have additional physical illnesses and to have less severe, non-psychotic, conditions. No differences were found in this respect between men and women although earlier studies had established that men are more reluctant than women to declare emotional symptoms and/or identify themselves as ill. The reasons why so many patients with psychiatric problems present with somatic symptoms are discussed below but the implication from this finding is that doctors and nurses who work with physically ill patients need to be especially vigilant when diagnosing suspected psychiatric disorder since the normal verbal cues may not be present.

The reasons why patients use somatization can be discussed by dividing the somatizers into three groups labelled here for convenience as 'deniers', 'disguisers' and 'don't knows'.

A fear of stigmatization frequently lies behind those who use denial since they do not wish to be thought of as having psychiatric difficulties. Such patients may therefore evade or even resent direct questions relating to their mental state and may even prove hostile to enquiries about their apparent physical complaints as well. Examination and diagnosis in such cases will call into play important skills with regard to interviewing techniques (see below) whilst helping the patient to feel less threatened. The aim in such cases is to try to build some sort of relationship of trust and then to allay the patient's often unrealistic anxieties with regard to treatment ('I'll be given tranquillizers'), diagnostic labelling ('I'll lose my job') and/or psychiatric referral ('I'll be sent to the madhouse'). This task may take several sessions before the patient is willing to open up and submit to more specific diagnostic probes.

Denial mechanisms can be found in any patient but they tend to be more common in males and in the middle-aged and elderly. Denial is also more common where the threat of social stigma is particularly pronounced as in the case of substance abuse, sexual dysfunction, marital disharmony. Denial may also occur as a result of the suspiciousness and paranoia sometimes seen in psychotic illnesses such as schizophrenia and in which case there may be the added complication of loss of insight. One might also include within the category of the 'deniers' a small group of patients who use dissociative mechanisms to translate underlying emotional and psychological experiences directly into physical complaints. The most common example of this use of somatization is the phenomenon of chronic psychogenic 'pain' often encountered in general medical settings.

The second group of somatizing patients (the 'disguisers') are those who recognize that they have a particular psychological or emotional problem and are willing for this to be diagnosed but who select alternative, physical labels to first engage the doctors' or nurses' attention. Such patients often believe that doctors and nurses are only interested in physical illness (a statement which is sometimes all too true) and they thus legitimize their reason for consultation by presenting trivial or unrelated physical problems. Real or simulated physical complaints are thus used as a 'ticket of admission' to gain access to the GP who, it is hoped, will then pick up on the other, more clearly emotional, cues emitted by the patient. Some patients obtain access to the GP by presenting 'through' another party, usually their children, a scenario reported as occurring prior to non-accidental injury.

There is a danger with the failure to detect underlying psychiatric disorder in such patients in that they may thus be encouraged to amplify their somatization either by making further consultations for the same complaint or by developing new (and potentially more interesting) complaints. If this process goes on for long there is a chance that the patient will eventually receive a specialist referral resulting in reinforcement of the chosen complaint and eventual expensive and potentially hazardous investigation. It is not surprising, given this mechanism, that a large proportion of persons presenting typically to gastro-intestinal, neurological or gynaecology clinics have somatized psychiatric disorders. The detection of psychiatric disorder in such patients is thus a major medical priority.

Particularly relevant for general practice are the third group of somatizers (the 'don't knows') who present early in the evolution of their condition and who have only a few symptoms. Such patients may not yet have recognized that they have an emotional or psychological problem particularly if they are developing a condition for the first time and/or if it is especially 'endogenous' in character (i.e. where the disorder itself appears to arise 'out of the blue' and has no readily identifiable recent precipitant). In general practice it is the patient with developing depression who is particularly likely to fall into this trap especially as many of the symptoms associated with depression are themselves quite 'physical' in nature (e.g. insomnia and fatigue). Within this group one might also include those with dual physical and psychiatric pathology who experience a deterioration in their existing physical complaints as a result of the development of disorders such as anxiety or depression.

DIAGNOSIS

In all cases in which psychiatric disorder is suspected, irrespective of whether or not the patient presents with somatic symptoms, the principals with regard to diagnosis are the same.

Observation

Look carefully at the patient's demeanour: notice how they're sitting or moving, the expression on their face and the tone of their voice. People communicate a considerable amount about themselves without actually speaking and much can be gained by affording time to sit and watch the patient as they recount their complaints. Depressed, stressed and anxious people often betray their deep unhappiness or emotional turmoil in their manner and appearance. Alcoholics may smell of alcohol or show physical symptoms of withdrawal. Patients with eating disorders may appear unnaturally thin – a factor disguised perhaps by their choice of bulky clothing. As regards the complaints themselves, it is often helpful to detach oneself for a moment from *what* the patient is saying and concentrate instead on *how* they're actually saying it. Those with psychotic disorders may exhibit thought disorder or talk to themselves in response to auditory hallucinations. Patients suffering with hypomania are not only irritable, eager or hyperactive but their talk may be fast and 'pressured' and difficult to follow through. Patients with dementia often show a tendency to ramble, to show signs of dysphasia and to have poor short-term memories. Those with toxic confusional states often have difficulty paying attention, are quickly distracted, confused, and may exhibit an aimless sort of restlessness such as repeated fiddling with their clothing. Much can thus be gained from engaging the patient in simple conversation and observing what is actually taking place.

A physical examination

Physical examination is a useful and important technique in dealing with those who present to doctors and nurses. Not only does this reassure patients who fear that their complaints might not be taken seriously but it may also yield important information with regard to their physical status which is of relevance not just to conditions such as sexual dysfunction, alcoholism or drug abuse. A significant proportion of psychiatric disorders are precipitated or caused by underlying physical disorders and it is all too easy to dismiss all physical complaints as 'psychiatric'.

Obtaining information from independent sources

An invaluable diagnostic technique is that of obtaining information from independent sources close to the patient. A patient's family and/or GP have the advantage of having known the patient a long time and having seen their deterioration. GPs also have a unique medical perspective in terms of the family functioning, the patient's social background and details of previous psychiatric difficulties which may have a bearing on the present condition. Relatives and the GP can provide crucial information with regard to illness course and can report whether there has been a change in behaviour or personality, whether this has been slow (as in dementia or some forms of schizophrenia) or fast (as in confusional states or affective disorder), and what their behaviour is like at home when not being observed. Sleep, appetite, weight, social withdrawal, loss of interest, memory, phobias, use of drugs and bizarre behaviour are all observable phenomena and will not have escaped those who know the patient well.

See the patient again

Psychiatric disorders often evolve slowly and reveal their true nature with time. If one is perplexed, diagnostically speaking, it is usually because one has insufficient information. There are a limited number of psychiatric conditions and it is remarkable how consistently such conditions manifest themselves in different patients despite obvious differences in terms of cultural background. In cases of doubt or uncertainty a repeat interview will often yield important diagnostic information. Repeat interviews can also be used to track and substantiate identified symptoms since duration and persistence are important diagnostic factors. Many people appear greatly upset or depressed immediately following some major upheaval but this does not indicate that they are necessarily diagnosable (or treatable) as suffering from a depressive or anxiety disorder. On the other hand a prolonged failure to 'get over' an event such as a bereavement (however 'understandable' the reaction itself might appear) may be due to the development of a psychiatric disorder whose identification and treatment will prove very effective when it comes to relief of symptoms such as sleep disturbance or inability to cope.

Mental state examination

Without doubt it is important always to conduct an examination of the patient's mental state. Knowledge of the basic symptoms and signs associated with each of the major conditions and some sort of experience in psychiatric interviewing are essential although neither is difficult to acquire and many non-psychiatrists make good and effective interviewers. Since psychiatric disorder is so commonly encountered in general medical patients, an examination of the patient's mental state should really form part of the standard medical clerking. It is often claimed that doctors do not have the time for routine psychiatric examinations of their patients. Such fears are usually unfounded and probably owe their existence to the kinds of over-long and highly detailed interviews taught to medical students in their psychiatric training. In reality, a considerable amount of diagnostic information can be obtained in a short space of time once one is familiar with the key symptoms and signs in each of the commoner disorders. In fact, early diagnosis of an underlying psychiatric disorder may, in the end, save valuable time by obviating unnecessary investigations, improving the patient's compliance with physical treatments and procedures and by relieving distress-related hypochondriacal concern.

In the light of these issues it is useful to consider the diagnosis of four conditions commonly encountered in medical settings: major depressive disorder, alcohol abuse, assessment of the self-harming patient and acute confusional states.

MAJOR DEPRESSIVE DISORDER

Depression is a common experience and a large proportion of persons with physical illnesses feel low and miserable. Only a proportion of them, however, have more severe and sustained disturbances of mood accompanied by the characteristic symptoms of appetite and weight change, insomnia with early morning waking, concentration impairment, suicidal thoughts, psychomotor retardation or agitation, morbid guilt or deprecating ideas of self, fatigue and an uncharacteristic loss of motivation, interest and ability in work or social activities. Each of these so-called 'associated' symptoms is itself quite common in general medical settings and the presence of one or another does not guarantee a diagnosis of treatable major depression. On the other hand the presence of five or more of these eight symptoms in association with a prolonged and sustained lowering of mood may well indicate that, whatever the original cause, a clinically significant depression has now intervened. The behavioural changes in depressed patients seldom escape the notice of friends or family and thus uncharacteristic changes in behaviour which cannot be attributed to other conditions (such as dementia) may well reflect this diagnosis. Depression is one of the commonest underlying diagnoses in those who present with physical complaints such as persistent pain for which a medical cause cannot be discovered. Exacerbation of existing complaints in those with chronic physical conditions may also herald an underlying depression. Finally, persons who abuse alcohol or drugs or who harm themselves or make attempts on their life may well be suffering from treatable depression, the diagnostic criteria for which will be the same as in the more straightforward cases usually seen in medical settings.

ALCOHOLISM

There has been considerable controversy as to when a person can be defined as an 'alcoholic'. In the past this term was restricted to those who showed signs of clear physical dependency such as early morning withdrawal symptoms ('the shakes'), tolerance to increasing amounts of alcohol, and reinstatement of full physical dependence on returning to drink after even long periods of abstinence. Patients with this degree of dependence, however, represent the malignant end of a spectrum of alcohol-related disorders whose diagnosis depends more upon the social impact of excessive alcohol consumption, which usually precedes physical problems by many years. For this reason medical thinking has veered strongly towards the notion of excess alcohol consumption as defined by 'at risk' and 'heavy' drinking. This is calculated on the basis of the number of units of alcohol consumed in the average week and in which half a pint of beer, a glass of wine or a measure of spirits are regarded as 1 unit. 'At risk' drinking is consumption in excess of 21 units per week for men and 14 units per week for women. 'Heavy' drinking is defined as 55 and 35 units per week for men and women respectively. Important social clues to the presence of excess alcohol use include early morning absenteeism, alcohol on the breath outside of normal drinking hours, decreasing competence at work and home, disrupted relationships, violence, and traffic and other offences. 'At risk' persons include those in catering and other 'at risk' professions, those working unsupervised hours, and those who work away from home and who are under stress. More subtle clues are contained in the CAGE questionnaire used widely and successfully in medical settings to detect those with 'at risk' levels of drinking:

1   Have you ever felt you ought to cut down on your drinking?
2   Have people annoyed you by criticizing your drinking?
3   Have you ever felt bad or guilty about your drinking?
4   Have you ever had a drink first thing in the morning to steady your nerves or get rid of a hangover?

DELIBERATE SELF-HARM AND SUICIDE

Self-harming behaviour is a common phenomenon in general medical settings and previous surveys return a figure of about 100,000 cases a year in the UK. Approximately 10 per cent of all acute medical admissions to hospital also fall into the self-poisoning category. However, only a small proportion of those who take overdoses are actually suffering from formal psychiatric disorder and/or are demonstrably suicidal in orientation. It is thus important to distinguish between 'low risk' patients (predominantly young females in whom there is little premeditation and small likelihood of repetition) and those in the 'high risk' category (including older, male, depressed patients with evidence of premeditation, continuing suicidal intent, physical illness, alcoholism, a family history of suicide, loneliness and recent loss). A third category of self-harming patient are the 'high risk' recidivists who are predominantly suffering from disorders of personality and have associated alcohol and drug abuse. Assessment of deliberate self-harm will pay special attention to evidence of (a) premeditation, (b) continuing suicidal intent, (c) demonstrable psychiatric disorder, (d) cognitive issues such as powerlessness and the degree of hope for the future and (d) the social circumstances including unemployment and/or other social or relationship problems which may not resolve. Premeditation is assessed by taking into consideration the degree of previous planning, efforts taken not to be discovered, carrying out the overdose in unfamiliar surroundings away from the home and prior declarations of intent such as suicide notes. In all cases of suspected or actual self-harm it is important not to shrink from the task of asking the patient directly whether they have thoughts of hopelessness, death or suicide as most patients in this position will readily accept help and will be willing to admit to feelings of desperation.

ACUTE CONFUSIONAL STATES

These are generated by some underlying cerebral or systemic medical disturbance the nature of which is not always clear and may be disguised because of the patient's inability to give a clear and coherent account of their complaints. By definition these disorders are usually of abrupt onset. They are also more likely to occur in those with reduced cerebral reserve (the elderly) and those undergoing surgery or suffering from identifiable physical illnesses. The marked restlessness, confusion, disorientation, insomnia and illusional misinterpretations and visual or tactile hallucinations in those with florid delirium are not hard to spot. Less florid cases tend to occur more commonly and diagnosis may be confused by the tendency for such disorders to fluctuate in intensity. A deterioration in behaviour towards the end of the day or at night with clear consciousness again in the morning is a suspicious sign. Repeated re-examination may be necessary to uncover the true diagnosis although, again, relatives' opinions with regard to abrupt and uncharacteristic changes in behaviour can also be helpful. In all cases one must search for the underlying medical cause beginning with possible intra-cerebral pathology and then proceeding to examine for specific systems failure in other parts of the body and/or metabolic endocrine or infective systemic disturbances. Alcohol and drug (including benzodiazepine) withdrawal states must also be considered since they may appear coincidentally in the post-operative period or shortly after admission in those with medical illnesses.

CONCLUSION

With practice, the diagnosis of these common conditions can be clarified within a few minutes of interview. The principal reason for not detecting these common conditions appears to be the failure to consider the possibility of their existence in the first place. It is hoped that the techniques described above will help to 'flag up' these conditions in the minds of those who will be working in predominantly non-psychiatric settings.

Chapter 10

Interviewing and counselling children and their families

Janice Kohler

Communicating with a child in a clinical context almost invariably means establishing rapport with his or her parents and may extend to contact with siblings, grandparents and a variety of other family members. Although it may be impossible to deal with a child in isolation, it is equally important not to confine the conversation to his parents and thus neglect the child's need for information and reassurance. Since childhood encompasses children of all ages from premature babies to school-leavers, the process of communication needs to be flexible and age-related.

THE DEVELOPMENT OF COMMUNICATION

Mothers naturally talk to their newborn babies and it is thought that the baby can discriminate between the sound of his own mother's voice and other women's voices by the tender age of ten days. By the age of two or three months, the baby will soon start babbling. This progresses to 'jargon', a series of sounds resembling normal speech but without meaning at first. The baby will imitate spoken sounds and natural noises and begin to relate spoken words to particular objects and events. The first spontaneous words, usually names of familiar objects, are uttered at around 12 to 15 months and these are gradually linked into two- or three-word phrases. Usually in the late third year, the child constructs and speaks sentences of several words with a simple grammatical structure.

The acquisition of language progresses simultaneously with the development of non-verbal communication. Sounds, gestures and body contact enable reciprocal communication of feelings and emotions between parent and child long before the appropriate words are learned. Young children are very sensitive to a stranger's facial expression, tone of voice or gestures, and may be frightened and uncooperative if these upset them.

In the clinical interview, some children as young as three or four years can participate verbally in discussions about their health, and older children should be considered the primary informant with parental support. Consultations all too often involve only the physician and the parents with contact between the doctor and child being limited to the physical examination.

THE FIRST INTERVIEW

When meeting any patient for the first time, and particularly a child, first impressions may influence the course of events. The child may already have sensed his parents' anxiety, he may be wary of strange surroundings, and if he has had to wait for any length of time, he may be fractious or hungry. There is nothing worse than starting a consultation with a family when each person is tense and anxious. Waiting must be kept to a minimum and plenty of distractions should be provided for the child in terms of toys and games. If their child is happy, most parents can relax too.

Many children are anxious about having to meet a stranger, and doctors may have been presented to them as figures of authority. White coats may frighten them further, perhaps because of previous contact with a dentist, and many paediatricians have abandoned their medical 'uniform'. This makes it all the more important that the doctor clearly introduces himself to the whole family so that they know immediately to whom they are speaking. A welcoming smile and quiet voice reassure the small child, and greeting him by name makes him feel special and included in the consultation.

Putting the child at ease

Allowing sufficient time for an initial interview is vital, so that the doctor, parent and child can establish rapport and become comfortable with each other before discussing the main purpose of the visit. Success in putting strangers at their ease is a skill which develops over years of practice and is a continuing challenge to the clinician. Children often carry a favourite toy with them and this can provide an instant topic of conversation. There should be a variety of interesting books and toys in the clinic or on the ward in which the doctor can interest the child. If the patient is too old for toys, appropriate seasonal questions, related to Christmas or summer holidays for example, can be useful, or enquiries as to what lessons are being missed at school. The doctor should be seated, so that he is not towering over the child, and at a 'safe' distance from the patient. Children are nervous if a strange person comes too close to them without warning.

Communicating with children is much more a process of establishing contact than an exchange of verbal content. This initial period of seemingly unstructured chatting with the child not only establishes communication but gives the doctor time to observe how the child behaves before any potentially threatening subjects are discussed or examinations undertaken. The way mother and child relate to one another may be pertinent to the medical problem with which the child has presented. If the doctor is clearly taking an interest in their child, most parents feel more relaxed and their confidence in the doctor's opinion grows.

The interview setting is important since a young child may be constantly distracted by surrounding activity on a busy ward for example, whereas the older child may be too embarrassed to discuss personal matters. Children are often regarded with less respect and sensitivity than adults and the need for privacy is overlooked. Even in a cubicle or consulting room, teenagers should not be expected to undress in front of their parents; a curtain or screen should be drawn round the examination couch.

Getting the child's view

Inviting the child to describe his problem may not produce such a detailed factual account as you would get from the parent, but his account may emphasize the importance of the condition to the child himself. Whereas a parent may explain that the child has had eczema for a number of years, the child may say 'I have a rash and everyone laughs at me at school'. Children mix with siblings or peers and their reactions have a profound effect on the patient. In the oncology clinic parents are concerned about details of treatment and long-term prognosis, whereas most of the children accept their disease and are only worried about returning to school with a bald head. Only by carefully and sensitively questioning the child can one understand the child's perspective on the problem.

The way in which a question is phrased can inhibit or indeed promote effective communication with a child. It is easy to be condescending or patronizing and a child will respond by being defensive or withdrawn. Although humour facilitates comfortable conversation, laughing at what a child says is only appropriate if he meant it to be funny. Clever remarks or jokes made aside to the parents may make a child uncomfortable.

It should be unnecessary advice to use simple language when talking to patients of any age, but medical people slip unintentionally into medical jargon. With young children the doctor needs to find out what words they use for various parts of the anatomy and normal bodily functions and then make the necessary enquiries without embarrassment or mirth. Avoiding the issue and simply asking 'how often does he go to the toilet?' leads to confusion and ambiguity.

Physical examinations

If the interview has been handled well, most children will cooperate with a physical examination provided every stage is carefully and unhurriedly explained in advance. Suddenly poking an autoscope into a child's ear will undoubtedly make him scream even if it does not hurt, whereas allowing him to play with the instrument or demonstrating its use on his mother first will often secure cooperation. The paediatrician John Agley taught 'If any child cries it is my fault' and, although not always true, it encourages the correct attitude in the physician. Occasionally it may be necessary to insist on examining an unwilling child, but not only are the physical signs almost impossible to elicit, it is a very distressing experience for the doctor, mother and child and erodes the confidence which has been carefully built up.

At the end of the interview, the doctor must explain his opinion and its implications to both the parent and child. Any investigations required can be simply explained and further details sent by post if necessary. If a kidney X-ray is needed, for example, the parents should know that an intravenous injection will be necessary so that they do not make false promises to the child that 'nothing will hurt, it's only a picture'. Most parents however, prefer to explain about the needle on the day of the test, so that the child does not have too much time to worry about it. Although the mother will be glad to know what a test entails, she will not thank the doctor if her child has sleepless nights for a month worrying about the injection!

Thus nothing should be said in the presence of even a young child which the mother would not be prepared to discuss openly. Even when they seem absorbed in a game of their own, children hear what is being said about them and may be worried.

FAMILIES WITH LONG-TERM MEDICAL PROBLEMS

Families who attend clinics regularly react quite differently from the newcomers. They quickly build up a relationship with doctors and nurses, especially if they see the same people each time. Even visits which involve painful procedures such as injections become routine and are accepted with little fuss by most children as long as familiar staff are involved. Young children quickly incorporate hospital visits into their lives and sometimes even assume that everyone goes regularly for blood tests. A new doctor who insists on using a different vein from which to take blood, however, may find much more resistance. Indeed children and their parents may become very dependent on clinic staff and may be quite upset when a favourite doctor or nurse leaves. It is important that they are advised of any changes in staffing which may affect them and introduced in advance to others involved in their care thus offering continuity.

As the relationship develops between the physician and the family over the months, or sometimes years, of clinic visits, many of the normal doctor/patient barriers are breached. This is normally a positive experience whereby the child is relaxed and the doctor enjoys seeing him again. However, it can lead to problems if the child feels he cannot upset the 'nice doctor' by complaining about his treatment or disease. Similarly the parents may be so grateful to the doctor for his help that they feel unable to voice their misgivings or frustrations.

THE ADOLESCENT WITH CHRONIC ILLNESS

Conversely older children become very wise as to how to please the doctor and keep the visit short, and may only tell him what he wants to know. The classic example is at the adolescent diabetic clinic where the waiting time is spent carefully filling in the last few weeks of the diabetic diary with normal values, perhaps with an occasional high or low number to add authenticity. The unwary junior doctor may accept the record as accurate and congratulate the youngster on his diabetic control, whereas the seasoned consultant is more likely to tactfully challenge the result.

Many teenagers rebel against their treatment, particularly if they find they can miss occasional tablets, for example, without immediate disastrous effects. It is a particularly difficult time for parents who have been naturally protective of a child with a chronic illness, and find it hard to delegate the responsibility for remembering medicines or diets to the adolescent, especially when they are not very reliable. Parents have to be helped to 'let go' and the youngsters counselled as to how to take over. Special clinics for teenagers with a particular disease, such as diabetes, can be helpful since the patients can meet and talk to others with similar problems and can gradually be invited to see the doctor or dietician without their parents if they wish. There may be personal matters which they wish to discuss in confidence without parental involvement. Similarly, weekend or summer camps for these groups of children help them to develop independence safely.

If a child is diagnosed as having a chronic disorder such as epilepsy or diabetes when very young, they need regular updating of age-appropriate information as they grow up. By the time they are teenagers they must fully understand the nature of their medical problem and the long-term implications. Quite apart from the practical importance of learning to live with a chronic illness, the young adult will feel angry and resentful if he suddenly discovers that he has not been told the whole story.

Deciding when a patient should be transferred to an adult clinic is not easy and may be an upsetting time for the youngster. It is usually appropriate for the paediatrician to look after him until he leaves school, but inevitably some patients mature faster than others and each must be considered individually. In some centres joint clinics are held by the paediatrician and adult physician during the transition period for patients with chronic disease, so that transfer is not so abrupt.

TALKING TO SIBLINGS

Children often experience mixed feelings about a sick brother or sister. They are naturally sorry to see him suffer but may also be envious of the extra attention he receives from the family. This becomes exaggerated if the illness is prolonged, and particularly if the sick child is hospitalized and one parent resides with him. Friends and relatives may shower gifts upon the ill child, seemingly ignoring the siblings who already feel deprived of attention.

Young children who feel rejected may exhibit behavioural changes, becoming withdrawn or regressing developmentally. Temper tantrums may occur and psychosomatic symptoms develop in older children. These are predictable responses and part of the medical team's responsibility to the sick child and his family is to help parents to anticipate such difficulties and to find ways of minimizing them. Siblings should be encouraged to visit the sick child in hospital and to find little tasks to do for him. Any special treats should be planned around all the children and parents should find time to spend with the siblings, even though they feel they need to devote themselves to the sick child.

Most children spend a large proportion of their waking hours in school, and teachers should be informed when families are disrupted by illness. They may then understand and be able to help unexpected behaviour in the siblings. Sometimes it is useful for these children to talk to the doctor or nurse on their own. It occasionally emerges that they are feeling guilty about their sibling's illness and wonder if they might in some way have caused it. They may worry that they too will become ill and need strong reassurance that this is not the case.

PREPARING CHILDREN FOR FRIGHTENING EXPERIENCES

We all fear the unknown and however unpleasant an inevitable experience may be, we feel more in control of the situation if we know what to expect. Children are no different, and once they suspect that some form of medical intervention is in store, they require explanations.

Many children's hospitals run a pre-admission programme for children awaiting surgery. The whole family are invited to visit the hospital a week or two prior to the operation so that at least the surroundings and staff uniforms are familiar. Booklets and videos are available, and the child can see some items of hospital equipment. Because it is so obvious to an adult, it is easy to forget to tell a child that he will have a general anaesthetic, and he may not know how to ask. It also helps to provide practical details such as the approximate size of the incision, or how many stitches might be needed, since if no indication is given the child will almost certainly imagine something far worse. Answering the unasked question is another skill required when working with children.

Play-acting difficult situations is useful for very young children. Putting a drip on dolly or holding the mask over teddy's face not only makes the frightening experience more mundane, but may also help the child to give vent to his own feelings of frustration or anger. Children who are carefully prepared tolerate unpleasant situations far better.

However carefully planned, children may still object violently when it comes to the point of intervention, and verbal communication becomes useless. Threats only inflame the situation: if a child is already hysterical whilst having a blood test, it does not help him to be told that mummy will go away if the noise continues. If the procedure is brief, like venesection, it is usually better to ignore any delaying tactics and gently but firmly complete the task. Having discovered that the experience was not really as bad as he anticipated, the child may be much less upset next time. Small 'incentives' for good behaviour may encourage cooperation but can be habit-forming and parents should be warned to be careful not to incite sibling jealousy nor to risk bankrupting themselves!

A star chart is a simple and effective way of encouraging desired behaviour. Each time a child has his injection without fuss, for example, or has a dry bed in the morning if he is enuretic, he sticks a star on the space for that day on the chart. This involves the child in his therapy and small children are delighted when they are congratulated on a row of stars. Once the good habit is established the chart becomes superfluous.

Breaking bad news

Most parents remember with great clarity the interview with the doctor who informed them that their child had a life-threatening or handicapping illness. Although they may not recall the content of the discussion, they can often describe in minute detail the room, the people present, the attitude of the doctor or the manner in which the news was imparted. Anticipatory grief starts from the moment the diagnosis is known, and its course may be influenced by the way in which the interview is handled.

Several studies suggest that parents value an open, sympathetic, direct and uninterrupted discussion of the diagnosis in private that allows sufficient time for them to absorb the news and seek clarification of certain points. Ideally both parents should be present, so that they can support each other and so that one parent does not have to relay information to the other. However, parents also want to be given results as soon as they are available and delays inevitably occur if both parents cannot be immediately located. As few staff as possible should be present, but it does help to include the ward sister or the doctor since they see the family on a daily basis and can reiterate and clarify what was said.

The amount of information which parents can absorb in their state of shock is variable but often small. It is best to stick to a few facts and to arrange a follow-up interview a day or two later. The most important information to convey is the name of the disorder, that the diagnosis is certain, what the implications of the diagnosis are, and the immediate plan in brief. If parents have been worried about their child for a long time, they are often relieved that the illness has been identified and is a recognized condition. As they pass on the news to family and friends, questions about the aetiology of the disease and the details of treatment emerge and require answers. Written information is a useful backup to discussion, and there are numerous booklets produced by support groups for patients with a variety of disorders. If insufficient information is provided many parents search public libraries for out-of-date medical texts and begin a quest for alternative approaches.

Involving the child

After the interview parents appreciate being left alone for a short while. They need time to weep in private, to comfort each other and to prepare themselves to face their child. Finding the right words is not easy, and some parents prefer the doctor to talk to their child. Both parents should be encouraged to accompany the doctor so that they can support each other and also to demonstrate that they and the medical team are in agreement, and working together to help the child. Whatever the child's age, he will sense his parents' sorrow and require some explanation. Withholding information from children seems to be unsuccessful in reducing their anxiety when something is so clearly amiss. If age-appropriate explanations are not forthcoming, children are prone to fantasize.

Older children may be resentful that their parents have been interviewed by the doctor on their own and quite reasonably want to know what has been said behind their backs. A few conciliatory words from the doctor may help, such as 'I felt I had to discuss your illness with your parents first, since it is a serious one. However we all agree that you are old enough to know what the problem is, and after all, it is your body we're talking about so we've come to explain what is going on'.

Just as the parents may have been relieved to have the disease named, so too the child may feel more in control when he knows what is wrong. A disease that everyone is afraid to talk about is much more frightening than one which can be named and discussed openly. However parents are often anxious about telling their child he has a disease such as cancer because of the negative connotations attached to the word. 'Cancer' often has no more meaning than tonsillitis to a child and if he will be attending a specialist clinic he is sure to hear the word sometime. Children have far more access to information nowadays and television programmes or publicity posters tell them about a wide range of life-threatening disorders. Not infrequently they hear other children at school talking about their illnesses. It is far preferable for it to have been fully discussed in an atmosphere of love and sensitivity within the family.

It is usually possible to be realistic and optimistic even about serious diseases. A child needs to know that he is very ill or he cannot be expected to tolerate unpleasant treatment, but he also needs to know that the long-term plan is to make him better or keep his symptoms under control. He must be given the opportunity to ask questions. These are usually limited to the immediate future – when he will go home, whether he can go swimming and similar concerns. Very few children explore the details of their illness at the first interview and death is rarely mentioned. However, they may well cross-examine their parents later and it is helpful if the parents have thought out what to say in advance so that they are not surprised into a rash reply. A truthful answer which leaves room for hope is best, such as 'Children do die of this illness, but we know you're having the best treatment and we're going to fight the disease together and keep you well'.

DEATH AND BEREAVEMENT

If the child's condition deteriorates because of progressive disease as in cystic fibrosis or muscular dystrophy, or if the cancer comes back despite aggressive treatment, there usually comes a time when it is clear that death is inevitable. The doctor may feel that it is inappropriate to continue with aggressive therapy, and that good palliative care should be instituted. Discussing this with the parents often brings back all the pain of the first interview when they were told he was ill, except that there is a degree of acceptance rather than shock. The family have already grieved for the healthy child they lost at the time of diagnosis.

Answering the unasked question is a skill required particularly when counselling parents for bereavement. Even if they do not ask, they need to know approximately how long their child might live. The duration of terminal care is variable and unpredictable, but a physician's estimate is the best guess available and helps the family to make appropriate plans. Parents also need to know how their child will die. Most experience suggests that when a child dies after a defined period of terminal illness, death can be made painfree and dignified. Unless one tries to discuss what may or may not happen, parents facing this situation usually imagine something far more traumatic and the fear of the moment of death may dominate and spoil their last few days with their child.

Children, too, should be given the opportunity to talk about death, although not all will wish to do so. Young children have no fear of death since they do not see it as permanent. By the age of around six years children understand that death involves physical harm to the body which is irreversible, and this concept may be consolidated by the loss of a family member or pet. From about the age of ten years, children evolve an adult understanding of death. Like adults, some children seem to know intuitively when they are going to die, but find it hard to talk about especially if their parents are trying to protect them from the knowledge of the inevitability of death. Children need time to put their lives in order and say goodbye, and it can be an enormous relief when death is openly discussed and the whole family can grieve together.

CONCLUSION

Communicating with children can be exciting and straightforward. It can also be frustrating and unrewarding. It is vital to create the right atmosphere to facilitate communication and to adopt an attitude of patience and respect towards each child. Children with a medical problem should not only be seen, but also heard.

SUGGESTED FURTHER READING

Kohler, J.A. and Radford, M. (1989) 'The dying child', in T. Burnes and J.H. Lacey (eds) *Psychological Management of the Physically Ill*, London: Churchill Livingstone.

Spinetta, J.J. and Deasy-Spinetta, P. (1981) *Living with Childhood Cancer*, St Louis: C.V. Mosby.

Vaughan, V. (1979) 'Developmental paediatrics', in W. Nelson (ed.) *Textbook of Paediatrics*, London: Saunders.

Woolley, H., Stein, A., Forrest, G.C. and Baum, J.D. (1989) 'Imparting the diagnosis of life threatening illness in children', *British Medical Journal*, 298: 1623–6.

Chapter 11

Interviewing the aggressive patient

Jeremy Coid

There are few members of the caring professions who work in everyday anticipation of violence towards them from their clients or patients. This was not always the case. Records from the last century show that violent behaviour was common among lunatics confined to the asylums where a custodial form of care prevailed. Felix Post, a psychiatrist who has now retired, described his experiences in the era before the introduction of phenothiazine medication when he had to be flanked by nurses on certain wards to protect him from patients who would bodily hurl themselves at him. The threat of violence may now be less common in psychiatric hospitals but the risk still remains within the Health Service, and violence may affect the lives of many professionals at some time in their career. For example, a study in Dundee found that one in every 25 of general practitioners' patients was potentially violent and estimated that threats of violence occur in one in every 500 consultations. In London the percentage of general practitioners assaulted rose from 0.3 per cent in a survey conducted in 1980, to 11 per cent in 1987.

Most assaults on doctors and nurses occur in the early stages of their careers. This is thought to reflect lack of experience but also the fact that junior staff have more contact with patients whilst seniors spend more time with administrative duties. Certain settings offer greater risk such as hospital casualty departments late at night and at weekends, locked wards in psychiatric hospitals, and prisons. Social workers appear to be more at risk from clients in their homes than in their own offices, but residential social workers in children's homes seem particularly at risk from their adolescent clients. Putting the situation in perspective, the rate of serious injury in the Health Service is thought to be twice as high as in the construction industry and five times as high as in the manufacturing industry. What is clear from these statistics is that all trainees in the caring professions require some training in the assessment and handling of potentially violent clients and the management of potentially violent incidents. Learning these skills would also appear to be most important at the early stages of their career when the risk is highest.

The purpose of this chapter is to enhance a trainee's skills to cope with a potentially violent individual during an interview. However, this is just one facet of the management of a violent person. The chapter does not set out to teach the reader how to restrain violent patients, 'break away' techniques, or go into the details of long-term management and treatment. Instead, the intention is to outline the basic principles, on the assumption that the reader will at some time have to carry out an interview with a patient who is aggressive, or else will suddenly be faced with aggression during the course of an interview. In some cases it may be wiser not to carry out an interview at all. It is hoped that this chapter will give some indication of how to recognize when this is the case.

The first part of the chapter examines the importance of recognizing and understanding our attitudes towards aggressive patients, evaluating the settings and resources necessary for the interview to take place, and the question of personal skills. This is essentially an examination of the basic principles when approaching the interview. The second part of the chapter presents a structured approach to the interview itself. This is derived from experience of working in settings where interviews with aggressive patients are more frequent, and will not necessarily be appropriate to all situations and all patients. It is hoped that this model can generalize to a situation where aggression arises unexpectedly. Aggressive individuals will be referred to as 'patients' throughout the chapter, but this is not with the intention of over-emphasizing a 'medical model' or excluding other professionals.

MANAGEMENT

Before discussing the process of interviewing, it is important to remember that the interview itself cannot be considered in isolation from the overall management of the aggressive patient. This chapter is orientated towards trainees who may not be at a stage where they have overall responsibility for the patient. Nevertheless, the interviewer does not merely require skills to cope with an aggressive individual but must also be able to understand why the patient is behaving aggressively in the first place by analysing the problem, assess what facilities and resources are needed to cope and whether any changes in organization are needed in the setting where the interview is taking place. Other colleagues and professionals from different disciplines may have to be consulted to facilitate a successful plan of action over the long term. Aggressive patients are usually complex with a multitude of problems besides those of threatening behaviour and poor anger control. If trainees are confronted regularly with these patients it is important to look carefully at their own management structure and position in the organization. Have they received adequate training? Are adequate facilities provided to cope with difficult patients? Does the trainee receive adequate supervision and personal support that is necessary in dealing with these difficult individuals? If the trainee is part of a team, is that team sufficiently organized and orientated towards putting an effective plan into operation, or is the interviewer left to cope with a difficult patient alone and without subsequent direction?

This chapter should help with difficult interviews in the short term, but if the answer to any of the above questions is in the negative then it is reasonable for the trainee to question whether he or she should be interviewing such patients at all. Unless junior members of staff are clear about the direction in which they are going, and about the overall management policy for such patients, their work will become increasingly stressful and demoralizing and it will be difficult and unsafe for them to work with this group of patients.

A highly disturbed, male, manic patient was admitted on a compulsory order of the Mental Health Act to a locked ward in a mental hospital. He had begun to show some improvement with medication, and three student nurses, who had recently started working on their first placement, were detailed to escort the patient in the hospital grounds for some exercise. The patient encountered a female patient near the sports field and began to abuse her verbally with a stream of obscenities. When reprimanded by one of the nurses, the patient immediately punched him in the face, knocking him to the ground. The other two grappled with the patient and wrestled him to the ground. The first nurse then kicked the patient. On return to the ward the patient did not complain and the nurses did not report the incident. However, it had been witnessed by a member of the public who did report it and the nurse was suspended.

This incident makes the point that aggression between clients and professionals is not necessarily always one-way, but is not presented for that reason. At the next multi-disciplinary team meeting some of the nursing staff roundly condemned their colleague's behaviour. However, it posed two important questions besides the professional qualities of the nurse concerned. First, what training had the three student nurses received in dealing with violent patients? Second, had it been a wise management decision to entrust unsupervised escorting duties of a disturbed patient to the three most inexperienced members of the clinical team?

PRECONCEIVED ATTITUDES

It is important to recognize that preformed and prejudged attitudes towards aggressive patients may make the situation worse and the interview more difficult. It is often forgotten that many aggressive patients are actually frightened themselves and that their aggression stems from overwhelming feelings of passivity and helplessness, with imagined fears of the destruction of their own self-esteem and sometimes their own physical selves. If staff respond by an increasingly authoritarian stance or by a counter-aggressive response this may increase the patient's feelings of helplessness and increase the risk of consequent aggression. In some circumstances it may be very necessary to use sufficient force to overwhelm a dangerous patient in a crisis. Where this is not the case, and particularly when embarking on an interview designed to reduce a patient's aggression, it is important to be aware of negative attitudes.

Negative attitudes may be shared by the staff team as a whole or held by the individual who has to carry out the interview. Conflicts between team members and shared fantasies about a patient's dangerousness can undermine the professional's ability to cope in an objective manner. Staff may have prejudices based on socio-economic, racial, ethnic, or educational aspects of the patient, leading to fantasies or stereotyped expectations of behaviour. Staff can also develop attitudes or feelings based on a single piece of history or behaviour before they have even seen the patient. If this leads them to expect the worst, then they may start to respond with increasing anxiety and anger, the subsequent clinical response on meeting the patient may be punitive, repressive, or neglecting, and this may actually provoke violence.

> A schizophrenic patient was readmitted after a further relapse of his illness on an emergency hospital order signed by his general practitioner and a social worker. On his first admission he had assaulted a nurse and had once served a term of imprisonment for a serious attack on a member of his family. A psychiatric report contained in his casenotes stated that should there be further violence in the future then a second opinion should be sought with a view to transfer to a maximum security hospital. Uncertain of the circumstances of the admission, additional nursing staff were sent to the receiving ward where there was considerable apprehension about his arrival. Upon arrival he was told that his belongings would be searched for weapons and that no aggression would be tolerated. He became angry and abusive and was immediately restrained and placed in a seclusion room where he remained for several days, receiving large doses of tranquillizing medication. He was later transferred in a drowsy state to a secure unit where medication was reduced and the patient remained well. He made steady progress and remained a 'model patient'.

It is important to evaluate what is known about the patient objectively and not attribute a 'larger than life' reputation for dangerousness when it is unwarranted. On the other hand, it is foolish to minimize obvious risks from information available and not take sensible precautions when they are required. A colleague who has interviewed a patient before and talks disparagingly about the trainee's anxiety may not only act in an insensitive manner, but may well have never touched on the patient's true underlying problems and aggression. Be wary of colleagues who proudly assert that they have a 'good' or 'special' relationship with a potentially dangerous patient. They may be bolstering their own self-esteem and colluding with the more negative features of the patient's psychopathology.

Inexperienced staff should not assume that there is always a right way of dealing with an aggressive patient. More experienced colleagues may well have better skills from practice, but it is not a hard and fast rule that they will always be more successful with every difficult encounter. If an interview gets into difficulties there may well be no 'right' way of behaving, just an ability to keep thinking until the next step is found, sometimes intuitively. Similarly, inexperienced interviewers should not feel that anxiety or fear are inappropriate reactions when confronted by these individuals, or that such feelings have to be suppressed at all costs. It is obvious that an interview cannot be conducted in a state of panic, but once experience is gained the feeling of anxiety in the presence of a difficult patient can be monitored carefully and these feelings can tell us what is going on and how the interview is progressing.

ASSESSING RESOURCES

If the reader has never considered what he or she would be if confronted with a potentially violent patient then it is perhaps time to do so. By rehearsing in one's mind how to deal with aggression you may find it easier to deal with the real thing. The first rule when approaching such an encounter is that no interview can be successful unless the interviewer feels confident. It is therefore important to consider what resources are available to feel confidence. Does the interviewer have sufficient personal experience and training to conduct such an interview? Has he/she been taught how to calm agitated patients, watched others doing it, or had the opportunity to sit in whilst a more experienced colleague interviews a difficult patient? The more personal experience the interviewer has already got the easier it will be to cope if aggression occurs unexpectedly. In addition, the more likely a professional is to encounter aggressive patients in their everyday working life then the more they will need this experience.

Has the reader ever looked at their office, ward, or general environment in which they work and considered what they would do if threatened or attacked? Could they escape if necessary? Could the alarm be raised if a patient got out of control? Would colleagues be aware of their whereabouts? Is the interview being conducted in a room far from colleagues if help were needed, or are interviews being carried out after colleagues have left and gone home for the evening? Do colleagues have contingency plans that would be put into operation in the event of a violent incident? If the answer to any of these is 'No', then the professional's confidence will inevitably be reduced and if they have to interview the patient then their effectiveness in controlling the situation may well be reduced with consequent risks to their safety.

In a situation where a home visit is contemplated, the professional has least control over the environment and may be at considerably more risk than in a hospital or institutional setting. It is in the patient's home where the professional is at greatest disadvantage. The patient has more control over the environment, and other persons may be present. It may be a completely unknown environment and if the patient's mental state is also unknown there is a need for considerably greater caution. The professional should decide whether it is really safe, whether certain factors in the purpose of the visit may actually be provocative in themselves, whether he should be accompanied, and even whether the visit is necessary. If difficulties are anticipated then the professional should be aware of exits in the vicinity. Colleagues should always be aware of when and where the professional visited.

OFFICE LAYOUT AND DESIGN

It is well worth paying careful attention to the details of the room in which the interview takes place. The patient needs to feel secure and relaxed as does the interviewer, who has to remain in control and not allow a potentially violent patient to dominate the space. The room should be the right size, not too large to the extent that the patient can readily get up and pace around. On the other hand, it can be a highly uncomfortable experience to interview a paranoid or threatening individual in close proximity within a cramped office. The fixtures and decorations should not be oppressive and should be conducive to relaxation. Potential weapons and missiles such as ornaments and heavy ashtrays should be removed. Remember, a freshly delivered hot cup of coffee from the waiting room vending machine should be drunk, with polite encouragement, before the interview commences.

Pay careful attention to the position of the chairs. It is inadvisable to sit face to face with an aggressive patient in a confronting or 'eyeball to eyeball' position. Sit roughly at 45 degrees or place the chairs where patient and interviewer can look at and away from each other comfortably without appearing evasive, shifty or confrontational. Some interviewers prefer a desk. This can be placed as a 'barrier' between patient and interviewer and may give a feeling of relief and protection, but this will also reduce the ability to make emotional contact and will reduce the amount of control over what is happening the other side. Placing the patient beside the desk allows the interview to be conducted at 45 degrees with more contact but lends a degree of formality to the procedure.

Choice of chairs is also highly important. It is preferable for the interviewer to have a slightly higher and harder chair than the patient, ideally without sides so that if it is necessary to get out of one's seat quickly it is easy to move sideways and does not appear as if the interviewer is coming at the patient. Offer the patient a softer, more comfortable, lower chair. If the reader tries this out by changing places it becomes clear how much more difficult it is to intimidate another person looking upwards from a soft base. It is therefore highly inadvisable to conduct an interview with the patient standing, a position from which it is easier to escalate towards violence. Always encourage the patient to sit or return to a seated position during the interview. It may be advisable to terminate the interview if the patient will not remain seated. One further point to remember is that many paranoid and agitated individuals feel more comfortable with a wall behind them.

Both interviewer and patient should be able to get to the door without blocking one another. This will allow the interviewer to escape if it becomes necessary and the patient to storm out in anger if he feels he has to without having to push the interviewer out of the way. In a working environment where aggressive patients or 'unknown quantities' are frequently encountered it is helpful to have an office with two doors at opposite corners. At least one should have an unbreakable window so that colleagues can check on one's safety without intruding or disrupting the interview. The door should not have a lock that can be operated from inside without a key and prevent rescue. The key itself should never be left in the lock. The door should also be outward opening to prevent barricading from within by an angry patient holding the interviewer hostage.

It may be advisable to have a 'panic' button placed in a reachable position for the interviewer and connected to a central point where colleagues can be alerted if difficulties occur. These are rarely used in most hospitals but offer staff the reassurance that help could be summoned if it became necessary.

HAVING COLLEAGUES PRESENT

When an interview cannot be avoided and where there is a real risk of assault from the patient then it would be foolish not to have others present. In these circumstances it is essential to have skilled and overwhelming force available to control the patient without injury. In less pressing situations it is still reasonable for professionals to set themselves a rule that they do not interview patients alone when they do not feel comfortable. A successful outcome can only be achieved if the interviewer feels confidence.

Choose carefully when having a colleague or colleagues present. A large male nurse sitting quietly in the room may make the interviewer feel more secure but sometimes can act as a focus for a patient's aggression. Some male patients can be handled without difficulty by a confident, female nurse adopting a challenging but motherly manner in a situation where a male would elicit frank hostility. On the other hand, this may be a provocative combination for a patient with a history of paranoid beliefs about women or a history of sexual assaults on adult females. At the same time, if there is to be more than one member of staff present it is important to establish beforehand who is in charge of the interview and whether there will be any interaction between staff so as not to confuse the patient.

> A male psychiatrist was called to see a disturbed prisoner in the segregation unit. He had been moved from another prison to a special unit for psychiatric observation of inmates thought to have mental health problems. He was currently serving a seven-year sentence for a brutal sexual assault on a woman and had a history of previous similar offences. He had been totally unable to conform and demonstrate acceptable behaviour in the other prison where he had spent most of his sentence in solitary confinement in their segregation unit. He only lasted a matter of hours on the assessment unit and was too disturbed and threatening to interview when first seen in his cell, the doctor having to be flanked in the doorway by four prison officers. He voluntarily accepted tranquillizing medication and requested next day to have a further interview. He appeared calm and was seen alone. He informed the doctor that he could not tolerate the presence of female staff in the assessment unit and went on to coldly inform him that he would assault him, inflicting as much damage as possible before officers could intervene, if he did not receive the doctor's word that transfer back to the original prison would be arranged.

This is an extreme and unusual case but demonstrates that exceptionally dangerous psychopaths and those with nothing to lose from their behaviour are capable of inflicting considerable injury if it suits their purpose. It had been a mistake to interview this particular individual without staff present in the room in view of what was already known about him. In the event, the interview had taken place with the prison officers a relatively short distance away in the corridor and the doctor had a radio controlled alarm attached to his belt. In the face of the prisoner's threats the doctor wisely conceded to the demands and terminated the interview quickly.

One additional advantage in having colleagues present is the prevention of the patient losing contact with reality and incorporating the interviewer into his bizarre beliefs. Some patients have a tenuous hold on reality as a result of acute psychosis or stress in an individual with an unstable personality. Their ideas may be influenced by early traumatic experiences. Delusions or hallucinations may establish a bizarre and frightening psychotic transference onto the interviewer who may be perceived quite differently or as someone else. Having a colleague present can give some relief to both patient and interviewer from this situation, especially if it is known to have been manifested on a previous occasion.

PATIENT–PROFESSIONAL INTERACTIONS

Having assessed the resources available, it is helpful to briefly consider what is happening during an interview. It is essential when carrying out the procedure with an aggressive patient that the interviewer maintains his sense of purpose and is not diverted from this by the patient. There are established patterns in which all professionals learn to behave towards their patients and clients during their training and in the behaviour that is expected in return. One observer believes that self-presentation takes place by what he calls a series of 'quasi-theatrical' performances in which there is a collusion between those who are interacting. Argyle has described 'rules' which regulate the coordination and sequence of events. It is only by adhering to these rules that the special professional–patient relationship can continue. This will allow the situation where doctors and nurses can touch and examine intimate parts of patients' bodies and where particularly sensitive questions can be asked within an interview. If the rules are broken, particularly in the situation where violence towards the professional is threatened, then the sequence of normal events is dislocated and the professional may no longer be able to continue. It is therefore important to be aware of and stick to these 'rules'.

Personal appearance and professional behaviour is obviously important in maintaining the professional–patient relationship. Correct appearance and dress with courtesy in manner, often with a degree of formality, helps to establish the interviewer's role and the standard of behaviour expected from the patient. Some interviewers may feel confident to use an informal manner and first names, but this should be judged carefully, particularly during the first encounter with a difficult patient. It is not always correct to assume that one is disadvantaged by sex, race, or physical size as it is not always possible to predict the response of an aggressive patient towards oneself. One patient may feel intimated by a larger, physically more powerful male interviewer whilst another may perceive it as a challenge and behave with greater hostility. Many female professionals feel disadvantaged, particularly in the face of a history of previous violence or hostility to women. On the other hand, some aggressives are remarkably 'gallant' towards female professionals, apologizing for the obscenities that inevitably slip out during the interview.

BODY LANGUAGE

There is an exchange of messages in all social interactions, many of which are conveyed and registered at an unconscious level. Non-verbal communication of emotions is largely innate, partly due to the direct effect of physiological states and partly to the development of social signals. Amongst animals, the adaptive purpose of non-verbal communication is to keep other members of the social group continuously informed about their inner states, but it also displays the level of dominance of one animal over another. Attitude towards others is demonstrated by the nature of gaze, the degree of proximity and posture. Dominance in relation to higher or lower social status can be partly communicated by the relative pattern of bodily relaxation and asymmetrical body posture, for example, when one person has one hand in pocket and is casually reclining in contrast to the other person. During the interview with an aggressive patient there is a subtle competition of signals which negotiate at the non-verbal level the precise relationship between the two persons, with many of the patient's signals effectively seeking to establish dominance over the interviewer. Some awareness of body language is important in gauging the interview's progress. For example, increasing dominance by the patient may be accompanied by increasing tension and immobility in the interviewer with submissive head lowered and rounded shoulders in marked contrast to the increasing upper limb movements and prolonged gazing of the patient. On the other hand, progressive relaxation in the posture of both may indicate progress towards a satisfactory outcome.

During the interview it is important to be aware of eye-to-eye gaze and this has been partly addressed already in the positioning of chairs. Prolonged staring may be perceived as a challenge by an aggressive patient, yet avoidance of eye-to-eye contact may be perceived as evasiveness or shiftiness. It is best to proceed somewhere in between, with regular but not prolonged glances at the patient, increasing the length and intensity of the gaze when making important points or expressing care and concern. Head lowered and rounded shoulder posture signals submission and can be demonstrated in response to angry outbursts from the patient. Alternating from the submissive position to a more upright and direct posture can allow the interviewer to 'ride' the fluctuating emotions of the patient during the early stages.

Another important aspect of body language is that it will convey powerful messages regarding the interviewer's attitude. Lack of concern is not only conveyed by what the interviewer says. This can lead to escalating disturbance if the patient feels he is getting no response. Apparent anger in the interviewer may also lead to retaliation. Empathy can be conveyed by leaning slightly towards the patient to express concern when he shows features indicating distress. Need for closeness will vary considerably between patients. Paranoid individuals will find this particularly difficult to tolerate. On the other hand, intoxicated patients will sometimes tolerate a closeness that would be quite unacceptable under normal conditions.

INNER PERCEPTIONS

Interviewing aggressive patients can be a highly stressful experience even for the most experienced professional. These individuals can create a range of different emotions and feelings in the interviewer, all of which are normal reactions and professionals should not feel embarrassed about them. It is important to be aware of these and monitor them as they may convey a considerable amount of information about the patient and with experience will help guide the interview.

Anger

It is essential to recognize anger and deal with this, avoiding provocation and responding to insults. On some occasions it may be acceptable to express anger towards a patient in a constructive manner – e.g. 'perhaps people behave like that towards you because you frighten them and they get angry towards you in return' – or as a means to set limits on unacceptable behaviour – 'I can't help you if you are going to keep shouting'. It may be more appropriate to divert the patient onto other topics which make him less angry during the difficult parts of the interview and return to more sensitive issues when his anger is under control.

Fear

An interviewer should not approach an aggressive patient with the belief that he or she should never be afraid to show fear and that it is essential to remain entirely calm and relaxed at all times. If it can be achieved this is fine, but it is usually not possible. Struggling with attempts to contain such emotions may give a misleading impression to the patient. Fear of an aggressive person is a natural response which can only be reduced by confidence in the interviewing setting and situation, one's own personal abilities, accompanied by increased knowledge and understanding of the patient. Increasing experience of successful interviews with aggressive individuals and the careful use of resources, such as having others present, can help reduce feelings of fear. However, one should not aim to eliminate all feelings of anxiety as they can help to measure how the interview is progressing. A sudden unexpected feeling of fear does not necessarily indicate a fault in the interviewer's technique or a serious failure of courage. It may be an important sign or even the only warning of impending violence.

> A junior doctor was interviewing a paranoid schizophrenic who had referred himself to a psychiatric emergency clinic. She had elicited his main complaints, his personal history, and many of the symptoms of his psychotic illness but felt that he was not revealing all his hallucinatory and delusional experiences. He asked her the occasional question about herself but otherwise was not particularly inappropriate or intrusive in his manner. As the interview progressed she became increasingly uncomfortable for no reason she could identify. Eventually she became increasingly fearful of the patient. Intuitively, she decided to stop the interview and leave the room, making a polite excuse. As she walked along the corridor from the interviewing room towards the nurses at the reception desk the patient followed her, came up quickly from behind, and punched her in the face, knocking her to the ground.

The doctor's intuition was not the result of what the patient said, but the unconscious registering of a series of non-verbal messages from the patient's body language and subtle changes in his manner and mood. These betrayed his growing hostility and violent intentions which were the result of his paranoid ideas, now incorporating the doctor. Leaving the interview room was clearly the only course of action in the face of this growing feeling of fear. If an interviewer suspects that a patient is deliberating on whether to carry out an assault there is no alternative.

Confusion

With a particularly difficult patient, when the interviewer appears to be getting nowhere, or with a patient who talks about distasteful, emotionally charged, or violent material for a prolonged period, the interviewer may gradually feel overcome with a sensation of mental numbness or confusion. It is as if the patient has overloaded the interviewer so he can no longer think clearly. In these circumstances it is important to observe a fixed time for the interview or to terminate at this point, if only for a break, if the interviewer feels unable to change the direction. Having a colleague present the next time may be helpful and it is advisable to discuss the management of such patients with a supervisor or colleague later to reassess that work is progressing in the right direction.

Fatigue

Interviews with aggressive patients are among the most tiring and emotionally draining of experiences, requiring a high level of concentration which must be maintained for longer than usual. It is undesirable to have a large caseload of such individuals or that the responsibility for these patients should always fall upon one member of the team. If there can be a coffee break then the time to take it is after seeing one of these patients.

THE INTERVIEW

It is hoped that this chapter has so far conveyed some understanding of the effects that aggressive patients can have on professionals and some of the precautions that need to be taken. However, many readers will not consider it is their professional role to even set out to conduct a formal interview with such a patient. In some working environments this may be difficult to avoid however. Because of the nature of the caring professions, individuals who present in an aggressive manner may be perceived as asking for help or may even have been referred for treatment of their aggression. The nature of the professional's role may then be to assess the patient and carry out a plan of management. It is therefore important that the interviewer maintains his or her professional role throughout, but is aware of the limitations of what can actually be offered. For example, hospitals are not providers of accommodation or money, social workers do not provide medication, etc. An aggressive patient may be exerting considerable pressure to get the professional to concede to his demands and yet may have officially presented for the purpose of obtaining the professional's help. The rest of the chapter suggests a model for approaching the interview itself. This can be divided into three stages:

Stage I. Assessment and calming the patient
(i)   Pre-interview assessment
(ii)   Personal introduction
(iii) Calming the patient
(iv)   Eliciting main problems

Stage II. History-taking and counselling
(i)   Re-evaluation of direction and purpose of interview
(ii)   Further clarification of main issues
(iii) Working through anger

Stage III. Formulation and termination
(i)   Formulate main problems for patient
(ii)   Agree on possible solutions
(iii) Termination

In presenting this model there are two necessary caveats. First, the model is intended to be flexible and readily modified to fit in with the professional model that the reader already applies as a result of his or her professional training – e.g. clinical-history-taking for the medically trained, social casework for social workers, nursing process for nursing staff, etc. Second, it should not be thought of as a rigid model that applies to every individual and situation. For example, with patients known to be dangerous or in a highly disturbed state it may be inadvisable to even attempt to proceed to the second stage. An interview incorporating Stage I and a shortened Stage III may be all that is possible. For readers who do not see their professional role as involving regular interviews with aggressive individuals, the various principles described below, rather than the three-stage framework itself, are likely to be of greater interest.

Stage I. Assessment and calming the patient

Before seeing any patient who is known to be aggressive it is essential to obtain as much objective information as possible from previous records and other sources. For example, a telephone call to another professional may explain why the person is creating a disturbance in the waiting room. This gives the interviewer time to assess his resources and decide on his strategy to deal with the patient. It is important to be aware of how the patient's attitude may have been influenced by what happened to him on arrival before the interview began. Has he been waiting long? Have other colleagues, receptionists, etc., treated him politely? This may have to be dealt with and discussed at some stage of the interview.

The patient's behaviour and demeanour should be observed before and during the personal introduction. For example, he may have made a threat to a colleague or banged his fists on the waiting-room wall. He may be intoxicated and it is sometimes necessary to ask these patients to return when sober. He may be too volatile and aroused for an interview to be conducted in safety.

Personal introduction is usually the first interaction and can profoundly influence the rest of the interview. This should be polite and formal if it is for the first time. It tells the patient who you are and what your role is in seeing them – e.g. 'Hello, I'm Dr—, I was asked by the nurse to come and see you because you appeared to be distressed. What can I do to help you?' Sometimes a patient may need to be told at an early stage that violent behaviour cannot be tolerated if they are to be helped. Some patients may be so disturbed they are unable to reply at first to the interviewer's questions and may have to be calmed and reassured before a formal interview can begin. Once the request is made for the patient to tell what is troubling them, their response is rather like the opening gambit of a chess game. A statement of distress or anger, even if the patient cannot explain the reason for their feelings, indicates a direction for further exploration. An immediate demand, such as drugs or a certain course of action from the interviewer such as 'I want you to telephone my wife and tell her I'm not mad!' warrants caution before proceeding further. It may be necessary to state the 'rules' – e.g. 'I'm not a doctor, I can't prescribe drugs'; 'Perhaps I need to know a bit more about you and your problems before I can decide to . . .'.

If the patient is angry and aroused they should be encouraged to sit and encouraged to remain seated if they wish to stand. Encourage the patient to try and relax and talk about their problems. It may be necessary to offer medication and even to ask the patient to have a 'walk around' outside of the interviewing room (not in front of the interviewer) to get control of their emotions if this is proving difficult. Do not interview with other persons present who are also angry or aroused as they may escalate the patient's anger further. It is usually best to see patients alone unless there is a caring relative or friend who is known to have a calming influence, or in the case of the patient who is afraid of the interviewer. Try and find out how the patient felt about coming. Doubts and fears about the interview itself and its outcome may be allayed at the outset, although no promises should be made before more information is obtained. Once the patient can be persuaded to explain what is making them angry, display empathy by expressing concern, paraphrasing if necessary what the patient has said and reflecting on the patient's feelings, e.g. 'Yes, I can see that it made you very angry'. Finally, try and discover what the aggression is directed towards. Is it a specific person who has enraged the patient or are they in a general state of anger that could be directed at anyone, including the interviewer?

Stage II. History-taking and counselling

If the patient's problems or general demeanour are beyond the interviewer's resources, then the interview should be terminated. At this stage the interviewer should be clear about the direction in which the interview will be going and its purpose. Most professionals will have a training in eliciting the necessary information for their professional role and at this stage the interviewer requires as much information as possible (or is practical in the circumstances) to move to the final stage. It may be necessary to go over the patient's presenting complaints, what brought them to the interview, and their current social situation, e.g. housing, relationships, employment, etc. The professional is attempting to understand the nature of the patient's aggressive behaviour and its origins. Their personal and family history may include violence and abuse from parental figures and family members, or the witnessing of violence between them. If it is possible to obtain information on the patient's upbringing and longitudinal development, including factors relating to their aggression and impulse control, this will help in formulating their problems and planning a course of action at the next stage.

During this second stage the interviewer may decide to counsel the patient and help with the immediate problem of his angry feelings. The aim is to gradually reduce the level of anger and arousal by getting him to express his feelings and frustrations in a controlled manner. This can be time-consuming and stressful. Some patients will visibly relax and settle as they begin to talk about their problems. Others become more volatile and angry when sensitive issues are touched upon. The interviewer may have to move away from these issues and then return to them according to the patient's mood. Many patients are genuinely afraid and confused by the feelings and emotions themselves. They may fear that they are 'going mad' or 'cracking up' and be reassured to learn that what they are experiencing are normal, if somewhat extreme, emotions expressed by everyone in stressful situations. For some patients the interviewer will act like a teacher, explaining to them what they are actually experiencing and the links between these emotions and the life events they have experienced. It is often very surprising for inexperienced professionals to discover that these links, which appear so obvious to the observer, are in fact totally absent from the cognition of many patients. This is typically seen in personality disordered patients or those from severely deprived back-grounds, particularly when they are under stress.

Maintaining control

Aggressive patients often try to change the 'rules' of the professional–client relationship. Much of the verbal expression and body language is effective in dominating the space around them and the persons within it. However, if the interviewer cannot maintain control of the situation the goals of the second and third stages of the interview cannot be met. The inter-viewer must maintain the boundaries between what is acceptable and what is not acceptable, and these have to be reaffirmed in various ways without provocative confrontation. As has already been explained, this can be done by telling the patient that violence cannot be toler-ated or that the interview cannot continue if the patient keeps shouting. It may also be done by inference, for example by reassuring the patient that his legal rights will not be taken away and that he therefore cannot be compulsorily detained because he is not mentally ill and is therefore legally responsible for all his actions. By inference, violence would then be dealt with by the law from which he will not have an excuse on the grounds of mental illness.

It is essential that both parties stick within the 'rules' of the professional–client relation-ship. It should also be a rule that once the interviewer begins to lose control, or feels increas-ingly dominated by the patient, that the interview is terminated. A situation should not be reached from which there may be no returning. Colleagues who have got into difficulties with their patients have described some of the following warning signs:

(i)   Frozen fearfulness – a progressive anxiety and fearfulness in the interviewer with loss of awareness and control over what is happening. It is important to remain flexible in one's thinking throughout the interview and to be able to keep thinking if things seem to be going wrong. It is best to leave the interview well before clarity of thought is lost.

(ii) Dehumanization. It is easier to assault someone who does not have normal, likeable, human qualities. Watch for indications that the patient is dehumanizing the interviewer – e.g. 'Social workers are all scum, they took my children away'; 'Call yourself a doctor, you're trash'; 'People who treat me like that deserve everything they get'. It may help to personalize oneself, sometimes giving certain details about oneself, rather than just the appearance of a characterless professional. But if the situation is escalating, then terminate the interview.

(iii) Failure to follow the patient's train of thought. With a very disturbed or psychotic patient this may be difficult anyway, but when it becomes increasingly frequent or is a deteriorating feature it may indicate that the patient is rapidly losing contact with reality or maybe deliberately withholding pieces of information and playing with the interviewer.

(iv) 'Point of no return'. A point can be reached in the interview when there is no possibility of returning to the normal rules of a professional–client relationship. It may become manifest with increasingly suggestive speech content, sexual innuendos, increasing physical proximity, and especially if the patient physically touches the interviewer in an inappropriate manner. This is the point to terminate.

Stage III. Formulation and termination

If the interviewer has helped decrease the patient's level of arousal and has collected sufficient information then a formulation can be made of the patient's main problems. It is important to give an explanation of your professional opinion in words he can understand. List the problems and potential solutions or alternative courses of action. This may not be easy with a patient who has set his mind on something else, who may not like the options or who tries to shift the interview back a phase. Be firm. Point out the limitations of what can be offered and resist going back over the same ground. It may be necessary to set in motion a specific plan of action – e.g. arrange urgent hospital admission, prescribe medication, etc. – which may make termination easier. If the patient is reluctant to leave because he has not achieved what he wanted it is still important to terminate firmly and not to be returned to the second stage. Make it clear what further follow up, if any, there will be. Explain politely but firmly that any new issues that the patient suddenly raises will have to be looked at next time.

> A young male patient had recently been released from prison having served a sentence for assault. He had a long history of violence, including two serious assaults on nurses during previous admissions. His consultant had diagnosed him as a psychopath and banned him from his ward on the grounds that psychiatry had nothing further to offer him. His imminent reappearance at the hospital emergency clinic was announced by a female patient who had briefly accommodated him in her flat and whom he had subsequently tried to strangle during sexual intercourse. She was now requesting admission herself to get away from him. He was 'interviewed' at the top of the hospital steps outside of the clinic by a junior doctor and nurse and requested to return in the afternoon to see a more senior member of staff. Later that day he was seen by a more experienced psychiatrist accompanied by a male nurse and social worker. The interview was extremely frightening for all three staff. The patient threatened them with violence if admission could not be arranged or money provided. At one stage the patient appeared to lose contact with reality. Little could be understood, but he seemed to think that he was back in prison and that one of the prisoners in the cell was making homosexual advances to him. He acted out a demonstration of how he would cut his throat and wrists, showing multiple scars from previous self-mutilating episodes. He then talked of persecutory voices and the delusional belief that he was a pop star. The psychiatrist barely maintained control of the interview but elicited sufficient information to decide that the patient was now psychotic, probably suffering from schizophrenia. He recommended medication in a long-acting injection which, to his surprise and relief, the patient readily accepted. The social worker obtained a place for him in a hostel for the homeless and the patient was offered a follow up appointment a week later. Over the next six weeks the patient showed a marked improvement in his attitude and demeanour. He was finally referred to another consultant in the Forensic Psychiatry department, by which time his mental state was much better.

This case illustrates many of the features already discussed in the chapter. To some extent the patient's reputation for dangerous behaviour was justified by previous behaviour. It was appropriate to interview him with more than one person present and the interview might have ended disastrously if the doctor had seen him alone. It should be remembered that when one department or agency refuses to accept responsibility for a difficult patient, that patient does not necessarily go away. Another department or agency may have to take up the responsibility instead. In this case, a shortened version of Stage II of the interview was employed as the patient was too volatile to attempt to calm by verbal means. The best that could be done was to offer medication. Issues of homelessness and destitution were equally important in the man's presentation as that of eliciting the symptoms of his psychotic illness which had been missed by other professionals. However, by tolerating this difficult interview the simple intervention of starting medication and finding accommodation had been so successful that by the time the forensic psychiatrist took over the patient's long-term management he stated that he could not see what 'all the fuss' had been about.

CONCLUSION

With experience and confidence it is possible to cope successfully with many aggressive individuals during an interview. Patients who behave aggressively are often profoundly distressed and later grateful for the opportunity to have shared their problems with a caring professional who is able to make sense of the chaos of their emotions and experiences. However, this is a stressful experience for a professional and risks should not be taken. It should be a rule that no aggressive patient is interviewed unless the professional feels confident about their own safety. Should control begin to slip away during the interview then it should be terminated.

One sobering aspect should always be accepted when working with these difficult individuals. The interviewer may have developed the necessary skills and confidence. In addition, he or she may have maintained control and coped with the patient throughout the interview, but this still may not be enough.

> A young woman of low IQ had done a considerable amount of damage to a hostel after a row with another resident and was told by staff to find accommodation elsewhere. Two hours later she presented at a psychiatric hospital demanding admission. She alternated between threats to the interviewing doctor and towards herself. Admission was refused and no amount of counselling could calm her when she could not get what she wanted. She refused an emergency placement in another hostel for the homeless. Finally, she stormed out of the interview and lay down in the road outside the hospital. When the police arrived, she jumped to her feet, punched one, and ripped the other's uniform. When it was established by the officers that she was not an in-patient and not considered by the doctor to be mentally ill she was arrested and taken away struggling and screaming. She was later charged with assault and criminal damage.

There should be a limit to the interviewer's expectations of what can be achieved. It is best to have simple goals for these difficult patients over the short term. The aggressive patient will often present multiple problems to the interviewer that cannot all be dealt with. Sometimes these will include a personal challenge to the professional, including the question of what their professional role entails. It is perhaps not surprising that the doctor in the example above felt considerable guilt for not preventing the arrest of this woman and subsequently debated with himself whether admission should have been arranged. By presenting at the hospital she had become a 'patient' and the doctor's 'role' was to help her. However, unless professionals have a realistic awareness of their personal limitations and those of the institution or organization they work for, then attempts to help aggressive patients will not be successful.

SUGGESTED FURTHER READING

Argyle, M. (1975) *Bodily Communications*, London: Methuen.

Breakwell, G. (1989) *Facing Physical Violence*, London: British Psychological Society and Routledge.

Davies, W. (1989) 'The prevention of assault on professional helpers', in K. Howells and C.R. Hollin (eds) *Clinical Approaches to Violence*, Chichester: John Wiley & Sons.

Dubin, W.R. (1989) 'The role of fantasies, countertransference, and psychological defences in patient violence', *Hospital and Community Psychiatry* 40: 1280–3.

Owens, R.G. and Ashcroft, J.B. (1985) *Violence: a Guide for the Caring Professions*, London: Croom Helm.

Roth, L.H. (1987) *Clinical Treatment of the Violent Person*, New York: Guilford Publications.

Chapter 12

Handling complaints

James Calnan

Clint Eastwood's career as an actor really took off when he starred in a series of Italian-made cowboy movies known as Spaghetti Westerns. In these movies he was 'The man with no name', the mysterious stranger who rode into a troubled town, single-handedly sorted out the 'bad-dies', collected his reward and rode off into the sunset chewing on the end of a cigarillo.

Many medics – and I include doctors, nurses, psychologists, radiographers, physics and so on under this term – believe complaints should be dealt with in a similar manner. Their attitude, based on this stereotyped Western hero, is that single-handedly and with proud independence they can sort out all problems and chase them away for good. Others believe that complaints should be ignored, for they will go away in time. Both attitudes are wrong. The variety of complaints that occur regularly in the practice of modern medicine, much of which relies on team work, are multifactorial in origin. Most have small beginnings and when something goes wrong every individual in the team is implicated.

Much of the experimental work on communication has been done with normal healthy volunteers. The trouble is that in illness we all change from rational clear-headed humans into irrational frightened patients, concerned solely with self-preservation because even with a purely physical illness the mind is affected. As a result patients forget what they have been told, refuse to accept disagreeable information and misunderstand even simple statements. They also criticize and complain. It is in these situations that every individual has a part to play. In my experience, those who make it their business to like the patients they meet and try to understand their problems and worries seldom encounter serious or even moderately serious complaints. The admonition 'Love thy neighbour' has never been more pertinent and the feeling is usually reciprocated. Grumbles are another matter. All too often they are golden opportunities to communicate essential information and cement friendships; one can only create friendship with patients by talking and sitting with them. And it doesn't come easily.

PREVENTION OF COMPLAINTS

Can one prevent complaints? Probably not all, but quite a large number can be averted. Half the battle is appreciating what the patient can reasonably expect from his or her medical attendants. Loss of any of these expectations may form the basis of a complaint. Here is my list of the eight most important items:

1   A certain amount of kindness. Aesop's observation is as true today as when written 2,500 years ago: 'No act of kindness, however small, is ever wasted'.
2   The necessary knowledge and ability to care for him in his illness, to advise and help him to make decisions with confidence. There is a fashionable view that a kind doctor can replace a competent doctor in modern high technology medicine. This is dangerous twaddle. Both are required, but kindness comes second. Even this judgement makes a basic assumption that kindness and cleverness could be mutually exclusive. Nothing could be further from the truth. Progressive medicine costs less in money and health than static or second-rate medicine; the patient and society expect nothing less.
3   Confidentiality in what he says to you and in his medical condition. Patients do not like their personal details talked about as though common knowledge.
4   Decorum in dress, behaviour and speech of doctors and nurses as a sign of their own self-respect, because in everyday life we use symbols to express the reality of a situation. Think of the significance of wearing a wedding ring; the trim uniform of nurses; the clean white coat of doctors. Patients expect their medical attendants to 'look the part'.
5   Interest in the patient's illness which you are expected to understand and take seriously.
6   Respect for him as an individual with a name and not merely a case number. Patients should always be addressed by their proper names, with title, and first names used when a relationship has been established.
7   A sense of trust which is possibly more important than affection.
8   A friendly environment. It is not difficult to say 'Good morning', nod, smile or look pleasant. A smile of welcome is always appreciated and the patient usually smiles back! A warm handshake is another greeting difficult to spurn, for politeness costs nothing and may bring rich dividends. A 'happy atmosphere' is recognized by patients more quickly than you might think.

COMMON CAUSES OF COMPLAINTS

What do patients do all day in hospital? Unless they are being investigated or undergoing actual treatment, they either listen to the radio, read the newspaper, talk to their neighbours or watch doctors, nurses and fellow patients for interest or drama. Most are bored and lonely. They miss their mates at work, a regular occupation, and have lost the freedom to do what they like. All this ferments complaints such as:

1   Not being given sufficient information about his condition and its management. Every

patient needs to know the diagnosis of his condition to tell his friends, for peace of mind and the removal of uncertainty. We know that patients only hear about 30 per cent of what is said at consultation and may retain even less. Hence the message has to be repeated frequently.

2   Lack of detail of what will be involved in certain investigations, a failure of communication that many identify as rudeness. With foreknowledge the indignity of lying naked in a cold room after a barium enema while the X-ray films are being developed becomes tolerable.

3   Pain which is unrelieved or unappreciated by the attending staff who are consequently thought 'unfeeling'.

4   Noise, either of voices of members of staff or other patients; snoring, repetitive sounds such as a dripping tap, or unexpected and unfamiliar sounds within the hospital ward.

5   Most patients wish to be treated with the respect of a valued client and hence will not accept uncertainty about the length of stay in hospital, equivocation about a date for return to work, or having to wait for such simple things as a bedpan.

6   In hospital the quality of food, being handled roughly and being treated as a simpleton because the ward routine is unfamiliar are also causes for grumbles.

All the above are preventable or correctable with little effort. What is needed is awareness. Many hospitals present patients with a brochure which sets out the ward routine, visiting times, how to obtain newspapers, books or toilet requisites, and the information that staff carry badges with their name, rank and function.

Serious complaints can come from nice people and invariably there is some foundation for them; they grow in size and importance – irrespective of the facts – the longer they are neglected. Indeed, a grouse matures into an official complaint with time. Arguments about complaints always have three sides – yours, mine and the facts – and these arguments may continue in the law courts as serious grievances. The greater the complaint, the greater the need for speedy action, particularly when several people are involved. It requires considerable self-control to listen to a patient's complaint that you consider unjustified, unnecessary and pernickety – particularly if accompanied by foul abuse – but it must be done. Although the majority of complaints are trivial, it can be difficult to distinguish the trivial from the serious unless the listener has an attentive ear.

DEALING WITH COMPLAINTS: GENERAL CONSIDERATIONS

The first time I visited New York in 1953 I stayed with Herb Conway, Senior Plastic Surgeon to the hospital on East 66th Street. In Britain we still had food rationing, much bomb damage, the post-war blues and quite a lot of poverty. In the USA, by contrast, food and money were plentiful, and emigrés were arriving daily. Many emigrés borrowed money to have their European faces altered to 'all American'. At that time there were said to be 600 plastic surgeons practising in the city and Conway had never been sued! One morning during my stay, a message came that a wound infection had been discovered in one such patient who was due to leave hospital the same day. Conway immediately went to see the patient, examined the wound, prescribed an antibiotic, and then sat down to talk to the patient and his wife. First he explained what had happened, reassured them that the result of the operation would not be spoilt, insisted that the patient stayed two more days but that he would not have to pay for this ('everything will be taken care of' – magic words). In ten minutes Conway had changed a worried couple into smiling, grateful friends. He also demonstrated the most important feature in dealing with all complaints: speed.

The effectiveness of a trouble-shooter depends on two things: reputation and reliability. A reputation for action, fairness, firmness, discipline, and the reliability for always being on the spot at the right time (or readily available) guarantee patient satisfaction. Consideration should be given to the following ten points:

1   Treat every complaint seriously and respectfully, however trivial it may seem at first. An informal method of communication is usually the most effective. A personal appearance is crucial, to allow the patient to ask questions and obtain authoritative answers. The person who persistently shuns confrontation communicates a vital and destructive message: fear. Complaints need action but the main need is to talk. Churchill once said that 'jaw, jaw is better than war, war' and recently a BBC reporter has updated this remark. Asked by a witness of brutal atrocities what could one individual do to help, Kate Adie replied simply, 'Talk about them. Let others know what is going on'.

2   Even if a complaint is expressed in fiery, abusive language, never be rude in return. Rudeness is unprofessional conduct. Keep calm and listen with friendliness, tolerance and kindliness. There are, after all, three possibilities in what the patient tells you. First, what is said is true and damaging, in which case you have to correct the fault immediately. Second, what is said is false and damaging, in which case you can sue – but this is rarely advisable. Third, what is said, whether true or false, is not damaging so why not make a friend rather than an enemy?

3   Treat every complaint as an emergency, to be dealt with expeditiously just as my friend Herb Conway did. Try to deal with the complaint that day if at all possible. It is better to tell the patient that you will return at a specific time to report progress rather than leaving the whole thing vague until tomorrow.

4   Never argue at the beginning because no battle is won by argument. Indeed, the only way to get the best of an argument is to avoid it. It is preferable to say that you will investigate fully and report back.

5   Listen attentively to the patient and his complaint (they are not the same!) Interrupt only for questions of clarification, then summarize in your own words and obtain the patient's agreement about the 'heart of the matter'. It has always struck me as curious that we teach students the importance of taking a detailed history before making a diagnosis, and then largely ignore the advice when dealing with complaints.

6   Investigate the complaint to the best of your ability. Question others. You may have to try to analyse the reasons for the complaint, before taking any action, and this requires concentration in a peaceful atmosphere. Talk to colleagues if necessary.

7   If you are in the wrong, say so. You should explain in simple, easily understandable terms how things went wrong and, if the patient is still not satisfied, offer to provide a second opinion. Make the explanation brief and to the point, so tell the truth. The liar is doubly damaged: by the truth he sought to disguise and by its exposure when the truth escapes. Do make an apology, but after the complaint has been investigated and

corrected, and make it sincerely. You may discover that there is a certain amount of satisfaction in apologizing. A grudging apology only makes things worse. To say 'I'm sorry' is not the same as saying 'I'm negligent'.

8   If the complaint is not directly your responsibility, say so. Tell the patient that you will find out who is responsible and report back, the same day if possible, and give some indication of when you will return, and thank the patient for drawing your attention to the complaint. It is often a good idea to return a few days later to ask if the patient is satisfied that the complaint has been dealt with adequately, because you too are interested in the outcome. This subtle form of flattery takes the heat out of a serious situation and implies that you owe a general responsibility for your institution.

9   Do point out the patient's right to complain and the procedure to follow in order to make a complaint official. For all serious complaints, whether relating to professional or non-professional matters, it is my practice to see the patient with a hospital administrator. The patient can make his complaint official and it will be reported to the health authority, if the patient so wishes. Few patients pursue the matter to that stage, but a proportion complain after they have left hospital even though little was said at the time. It should be part of the good practice of medicine to be alert to the signals of discontent and uncover them early because so often all that is required is ten minutes listening and talking; and this is better done at the time and not six months later when a letter of complaint is received.

10   Remember to thank the patient for having the courage to bring the complaint to your notice. When you can agree that a fair solution has been achieved, say openly that the matter is now closed. No stigma should be attached to any patient who has a genuine complaint and it is your duty to ensure that the patient is not labelled 'uncooperative'. The basis of good morale in patients and staff – whether in a hospital ward, out-patient clinic or GP surgery – is undoubtedly the free and easy flow of information by word of mouth. What begins as a routine ('Good morning. How are you today?') becomes a habit. A habit becomes a skill and a skill spreads confidence all round. Moreover the habit of saying 'Good morning' means that your patients are likely to become friends, whereas without the civilities they could easily become strangers.

THE MANAGEMENT OF COMPLAINT: FIVE LOGICAL STEPS

There are many methods for dealing with complaints but it is wise to follow a logical step-by-step approach.

1   *The pre-approach.* Learn all you can before seeing the patient and start immediately. Now is the time to judge whether the complaint is likely to be serious or trivial, and whether it can be classified as professional or general (non-professional). In all instances of complaints about professional competence or ability, a written record must be made and everyone involved must be informed. It is also wise to warn your superiors. In composing a written report brevity is an advantage because short reports are usually easier to follow. Current teaching is to 'count words' but better advice is to

'weigh words' because the right word that conveys the condition you wish to describe is really what is required.

2   *The approach.* Introduce yourself and try to choose a quiet place in which to interview the patient, and sit down with him. Listen to what he says, ask questions and make notes openly; there is no need to be furtive. A few quick notes in the patient's records at the time of interview are worth more than a lengthy report composed later. They may also carry more weight in a court of law. Tangible and relevant facts such as the pulse rate, blood pressure and so on should be recorded as well as the intangibles such as a sense of humour, gloomy outlook or boastfulness which can depict the patient's personality. Events should be recorded in sequence and the thread of the narrative be unbroken. The writer's opinion and argument come at the end, not interposed throughout.

3   *The presentation.* Summarize what the patient has said and your interpretation of this, in clear language. Be objective. In complicated cases it may not be possible to summarize the patient's statements immediately. It is then better to retire to think and return later.

4   *Dealing with the complaint.* Investigate in detail to uncover the facts and so discover a solution. Often this cannot be done in a hurry, which is not the same as dawdling, simply because there may be many people to interview. Where serious medical negligence is alleged the average time for the case to come to court is four years. Even a seven-year wait is not uncommon. For the majority of general complaints a period of one day to one month may be a reasonable delay.

5   *The close.* Discuss with the patient and others what can be done, but try to allow the patient to decide on the plan of action so that he becomes involved in the outcome. Ask if he is satisfied with the plan; if not, go over the grounds for complaint again. Finally, express gratitude to him for drawing your attention to the complaint.

Most faults in dealing with complaints are acts of omission: not listening to the complainant, not clarifying or defining the complaint, not being sympathetic or attentive. But some faults are less excusable acts, such as blaming others, doing nothing, denying that anything is wrong or covering up errors. If the trust of patients is to be preserved, complaints must be dealt with quickly and even-handedly. It is the duty of everyone looking after patients to be aware of the possibility of complaints and to develop the necessary skills to allay them. Some plaintiffs go to court with the expressed desire to discover 'exactly what went wrong'. In these instances an explanation in detail, and balanced arguments, may well decrease the amount of litigation. At least there is that possibility, in contrast to cases brought by those who seek revenge or monetary gain.

THE COMPLAINT OF PROFESSIONAL NEGLIGENCE

If you are a doctor and your patient accuses you of negligence in the management of his illness, this is a serious complaint. It is a life-threatening situation (yours) and demands immediate action. You must do three things:

1   Let your medical defence society know of the accusation by first-class post. Write a

précis of your side of the story, photocopy and send copies of all relevant documents: the patient's case record, lab reports, and all letters. Keep copies for yourself (you may have to keep them for seven years or even longer!). You will receive a helpful reply from a named individual and probably instructions on what to do next. Reply by return of post whenever possible; this is not just courtesy but a necessary speediness which allows the defence society to measure how the whole event will turn out. Not all cases go to court, so be grateful.

2   Inform your chief and ask the most senior colleague you can find to take over the patient's day-to-day management. Introduce him to your patient and explain that since the patient has lost confidence in you Dr X will look after him meanwhile. Say that you're sorry about the turn of events but that you have every confidence in Dr X. Say no more and do not argue. If the patient would like another opinion on his condition, arrange this too. Make sure that Dr X follows up your patient later. In my experience, once things get this far, it is better for all that the patient continues with Dr X and is not returned to you, irrespective of whether the case goes to court or not. Clinical medicine relies on trust between patient and doctor. Even then life can be difficult enough but without trust on both sides the contract becomes impossible.

3   Let the hospital administrator know of the accusation of negligence because, commonly, a claim may be made against the hospital or health authority as well as against the doctor. The administrator will ask for a report from you and may well commandeer the patient's records (hence the need to get hold of them first).

If you are not a doctor, it is wise to follow the advice above and contact your own professional advisers and insurers. No one is immune from allegations of professional negligence or incompetence. Frequently, of course, the complaint is made after the patient has left your care and the first sign of trouble is a solicitor's letter at breakfast. There is no need to panic but delay is detrimental to you. Sadly, the number of allegations has continued to increase – perhaps as patients' expectations increase – and damages awarded in the Law Courts have multiplied. As a result medical defence subscriptions have moved from 0.1 per cent of a junior doctor's income in 1953 to 7 per cent in 1988! Reading through the Annual Report of any defence society is salutary, for many of the cases were preventable and should never have reached the Law.

SUGGESTED FURTHER READING

Calnan, J. (1983) *Talking with Patients*, London: Heinemann.
Duncan, A.S., Dunstan, G.R. and Welbourn, R.B. (1981) *Dictionary of Medical Ethics*, London: Darton, Longman & Todd.
Hawkins, C. (1985) *Mishap or Malpractice?*, Oxford: Blackwell.
Mason, J.K. and Smith, R.A.M. (1987) *Law and Medical Ethics* 2nd ed, London: Butterworths.

Chapter 13

Using cognitive-behavioural techniques

Robert Newell

INTRODUCTION

Cognitive-behaviour therapy (CBT) is now the most extensively investigated and empirically supported of psychological interventions for a wide range of client/patient difficulties. In the past decade, there has been an enormous proliferation of research studies and the ambit of CBT has greatly widened from its original focus on the focal anxieties (phobias and obsessive-compulsive disorders). Although CBT is now the treatment of choice for these complaints, cognitive-behavioural interventions are widely used and accepted in the treatment of eating disorders, disorders of habit, marital and sexual problems and diverse medical complaints, notably chronic pain.

This chapter attempts to introduce the reader without specialist knowledge of psychological therapies to the general framework of CBT. The notion of CBT as something done by specialist psychologists is outdated. Numerous studies show that other health care professionals, with appropriate training, deliver such treatment with equal effect. In particular, psychiatric nurses with post-registration training in CBT (Nurse Therapists) have gained wide acceptance in the field, and multidisciplinary courses for doctors, social workers and occupational therapists have also been created.

By the end of this chapter, the reader should not only have an overview of the possible uses of cognitive-behavioural interventions but, more importantly, should feel able to begin the use of these interventions with a few clients during the course of a hospital or general practice consultation.

GENERAL STRATEGIES IN COGNITIVE-BEHAVIOURAL INTERVIEWING

Compliance with medical instruction

All interviews contain information and emotion. Additionally, the required outcome of an interview, for the clinician, is behaviour and attitude change on the part of the client. However, compliance with even very simple and non-threatening instructions (e.g. following an antibiotic regimen) is often poor. Cognitive-behavioural therapists have therefore come to concentrate on the interview process in some detail, in order to ensure effective information transmission and instruction compliance, often drawing on the work of social and cognitive psychologists. Most therapists would agree that effective interviewing should adhere to the following schema.

Set induction

Following appropriate introduction, the clinician should outline the aims, content and duration of the interview, so as to decrease anxiety and to allow the client to maximize the use of their attention, thus setting the context in which learning will be most likely to occur.

Information transmission – presentation and transfer

For compliance with treatment instructions to happen, information needs to be retained by the client. Whilst always following patient cues where appropriate, the clinician should attempt to maintain a logical sequence, and to proceed from the general to the specific. Again, this will make least demands on client attention, and, where information is presented by the clinician, will aid in comprehension by allowing both the client and the clinician to form logical connections between pieces of information, aiding recall.

The clinician should proceed from open to closed questions. As well as being less threatening for the client, open questions allow the client a variety of responses which the clinician then scans in order to select more specific questions which are required to clinch the detail which is central to behavioural assessment. Furthermore, this funnelling sequence gives client and clinician a general context to aid recall of specific information, both at interview and subsequently.

The clinician will, wherever possible, offer advice by Socratic rather than didactic means, guiding the patient towards a statement of what they should do, which also reflects the most appropriate option in line with the cognitive-behavioural formulation of their difficulties. Not only will the option appear more attractive to the client as a result of their involvement in the process, but the process is a kind of rehearsal by the patient which will render the information more salient in memory.

Information transmission – rehearsal and transfer

Cognitive, verbal and behaviour rehearsal are all powerful aids to recall. The clinician will allow frequent opportunities for rehearsal by repeated summarizing of both the client's information (allowing correction and elaboration) and any instruction the clinician may have offered. Paraphrasing by the clinician serves the same function, but additionally aids retention by allowing the formation of differing storage possibilities in memory. Inviting summaries and paraphrases from the client is a further similar tactic, with the additional advantage, where information has been given by the clinicians, of offering a check that comprehension has occurred. It should be noted that these tactics also convey clinician understanding, interest and concern to the client, not only cementing the therapeutic relationship, but also, in consequence, increasing the likelihood of client compliance with the instruction offered.

Behavioural rehearsal in the clinic, where possible, is extremely potent in inducing retention and compliance. Where such rehearsal is impractical, a detailed talk-through by the client of the behaviour to be performed is an excellent substitute. Both these tactics allow opportunities for the elucidation of any misunderstandings and the solving of particular potential difficulties.

Closure

Apart from routine arrangements for further meetings and eliciting from the client their feelings about the interview, the close of the session should be used for final reinforcement, summaries, paraphrases and rehearsals since the most recent events are the best recalled. The likelihood of retention and compliance is thus maximized.

PROGRESS CHECKLIST 1

General strategies in behavioural interviewing

Set induction

   Aims, content, duration

Information transmission – presentation and transfer

   reinforcement
   logical sequence of questioning
   general to the specific
   open to closed questions
   scanning through information from open questions
   clinch the detail by closed questions
   funnelling

Socratic rather than didactic discourse
(get the client to advise him/herself)

Information transmission – rehearsal and transfer

cognitive, verbal and behavioural rehearsal
summarizing
paraphrasing
summaries and paraphrases from the client
talk-through

Closure

reinforcement, summaries, paraphrases and rehearsals

PRACTICAL EXAMPLE 1

Compliance with treatment instructions

Doctor: Thank you for coming, Mrs Smith. Now over the next ten minutes, I am hoping to give you some initial advice regarding the management of your diabetes, and by the end of the session I hope we will have agreed that you will start to test your own urine. I also hope there will be time to answer any specific questions you have and to agree to meet again. . . . [**Set induction**]

Patient: It all seems so complicated. I am not sure that I'll be able to manage it.

Doctor: Yes, it can seem very worrying and difficult, particularly to begin with. [**Paraphrasing**] Can you tell me what you think the main difficulty might be? [**Open question**]

Patient: I think . . . managing the readings.

Doctor: What bit in particular of doing the readings? [**Funnelling to the specific**]. . . .
How do you think you might manage the testing in your own home? [**Encouraging client self-advice and competence**]. . . .
Just run through in your mind how you're going to do the tests at home, then tell me aloud. [**Cognitive and verbal rehearsal**]

Patient: Well, I'm going to. . . .

Doctor: That's an excellent description of how the testing should go. [**Specific reinforcement**] Let me now just summarize [**Summarizing**], before I ask you to actually have a go at it on the ward. [**Behavioural rehearsal**]. . . .

Doctor: And could you just summarize what we've decided [**Inviting summary**], and give me a detailed run through of what you're going to be doing between now and when we meet again? [**Talk-through and rehearsal at closure**]. . . .

Doctor: Excellent. Thanks for talking to me and working so hard. We are agreed we'll meet again tomorrow so as to discuss your progress. [**Final reinforcement and future planning**]

The practical example given demonstrates most of the techniques described in context. Although it is a highly stylized interview description (for the sake of brevity), it should show that eliciting and delivering information in a systematized way need not be an unnatural or time-consuming affair. Furthermore, much of the content of the interview might need to take place in any interview of its kind. The issue here is to be aware of the potential for such content to increase the efficiency of the process. Thus, rehearsal is not merely necessary to gain task skill, but is an opportunity for cognitive and verbal rehearsal of later performances, and reinforcement, with the aim of increasing compliance. Similarly, most clients can offer some account of what they think should be done in many medical circumstances. For the clinician to encourage this, with appropriate redirection, takes little more time than telling the client directly but increases the likelihood that the message will be understood and acted upon.

COGNITIVE-BEHAVIOURAL ASSESSMENT AND EXPOSURE ADVICE

Fear of medical intervention

Patients often find medical interventions frightening. Although in many cases this is both a moderate and appropriate fear, which the patient can overcome with simple reassurance and a supportive manner from the clinician, a number of patients find their fears so great that they avoid treatment, or certain components of treatment, completely. If they do enter treatment, their compliance is sporadic, because of fear and poor understanding of instruction owing to intervening anxiety. Apart from fear of medical interventions, clients may also fear illness (especially cancer) so greatly that they fail to seek appropriate testing or treatment if they notice something amiss. Both fear of medical treatment and fear of illness contribute to clients arriving for treatment when a complaint is already in an advanced state.

In such clients, the response to fear of illness or intervention is sufficiently severe to be regarded as phobic, and the appropriate intervention (which will ultimately save clinical time and resources) is exposure treatment, a cognitive-behavioural intervention involving advice to the client to confront the feared situations in a systematic fashion, capitalizing on the process of habituation.

Accurate, detailed and precise assessment which renders explicit those behaviours, cognitions and sensations which are problematic to the client is a prerequisite of effective cognitive-behavioural intervention. The scheme given below represents one model of behavioural assessment. As was noted in the previous section, much of the information might be required as part of a standard medical or nursing consultation; the issue is to use the information to aid in delivering appropriate advice which will reduce the client's fear.

Cognitive-behavioural assessment

After asking the client to describe the main difficulty in general terms, the clinician elicits the following information.

Autonomic

Does the client experience physical symptoms of anxiety before, during or after the feared situation? Is there diminution of anxiety once the feared situation has passed?

Behavioural

What does the patient do immediately before, during and after problem episodes? Here the clinician is looking primarily for precautionary measures, avoidances, reassurance-seeking, attempts to enlist the help of others. Who else is present? Do problem episodes only occur when particular persons are present?

What are the physical characteristics of the environment? Does the problem begin only in certain environments (i.e. are there environmental triggers to the problem episodes?)

The key question forms here are:

how long does an episode last?
how often does an episode occur?
when does an episode occur (day? time of day?)?
how severe are the episodes in differing circumstances?
how long ago was the last episode?

Cognitive

What thoughts and images pass through the client's mind immediately before, during and after a problem episode? In particular, does the client:

predict negative outcomes (e.g. pain, fear, fainting)
predict adverse responses from others
remember previous problem episodes
pretend they can avoid the current problem episode
imagine the current episode has passed
rehearse previous non-coping thinking patterns
overemphasize negative aspects of the episode
interpret physical symptoms as signs of impending doom?

In addition to the above, general information is sought regarding onset and fluctuations of the complaint. Here, the clinician is chiefly searching for information regarding times when the client has been able to utilize his/her own coping tactics to overcome the problem. These tactics may form the basis of the clinician's later advice.

Goals

By agreeing goals, the client is more likely to see the usefulness of treatment and to comply.

PROGRESS CHECKLIST 2

Cognitive-behavioural assessment

Autonomic

Physical symptoms of anxiety – before, during, after feared episode?
Anxiety relief – after?

Behavioural

Before, during, after episode?
Key questions:
   how long?
   how often?
   when?
   how severe?
   how long ago?

Cognitive

Before, during, after episode?
   prediction of:
   negative outcomes
   adverse responses from others
   memory of previous episodes
   pretence of avoidance
   imagining current episode has passed
   rehearsing previous non-coping thinking patterns
   overemphasizing negative aspects of the episode
   interpreting physical symptoms as signs of impending doom?

Onset

Fluctuations

Goals

Exposure advice

A careful explanation of the proposed intervention will enable the client to give consent and maximize the likelihood of compliance with treatment. In general terms, the patient is likely to learn a number of specific coping tactics. For the client suffering anxiety, this will always involve exposure to the fear-evoking situations, whether these be external, as in the case of phobias, or internal, as in the case of general anxiety based on misinterpretation of bodily stimuli and many illness phobias.

To be effective, rationale-giving should involve the following components:

1   *general description* of how intervention works (e.g. habituation – anxiety reduction as a normal bodily process over time provided the client enters and remains in the feared situation for sufficient time to allow such reduction to occur. Role of avoidance and escape in maintaining anxiety by preventing the client from experiencing anxiety reduction in the problem situations)
2   *specific description* of what the client will be required to do (e.g. an injection phobic might be asked to begin by looking at pictures of others having injections, move on to handling needles and syringes, before attempting to have an injection), emphasizing the stepwise nature of treatment, with the client gradually progressing from simple to difficult tasks as competence and confidence grow
3   *collaborative nature of treatment,* in which the client and clinician negotiate each step
4   *need for commitment and likelihood of some discomfort* in the early stages, but set into the context of the discomfort the client has already endured
5   *need to enlist others* (friends, family members, other staff) to help in treatment
6   *likely positive outcome,* and short duration of treatment
7   *planning of specific tasks* to be performed by the client (perhaps with aid and supervision) between now and next meeting. Relevance of these to goal achievement.

PROGRESS CHECKLIST 3

Exposure advice

general description
specific description
collaborative nature of treatment
need for commitment
need to enlist others
likely positive outcome
planning of specific, relevant tasks

Once again, this advice need not be time-consuming, and much successful treatment has been conducted on a largely self-help basis. In the practical example given below, an injection phobic, who has refused necessary blood tests on several occasions, because of fear of pain and of fainting, has agreed to attempt to solve her difficulty, in order to have tests necessary during her pregnancy. An obstetric registrar explains the nature of treatment. Again the example given is highly stylized, and in real life would include questions from the client and recapping by the doctor. Even so, advice of the kind detailed here can be given within about five minutes. The issue is to give the advice clearly and effectively.

PRACTICAL EXAMPLE 2

Fear of medical intervention

Doctor: Well, Mrs Smith, I'm really very glad you've decided to have a go at overcoming your fear of injections. I'm sure you've made the right decision. [**Reinforcement and attribution of positive attitudes, so increasing likelihood of compliance**]. Now I'd like to run over what this treatment involves. In general terms, as you know, we tend to get used to even quite frightening things if we do them long enough and often enough – like doing examinations and interviews, for instance.

Treatment works in the same way, cashing in on this natural ability of the body to get used to fears in this way, and so we encourage you to confront the very thing that you fear and to stay with it until the fear comes down. Much of this work you'll do away from here, as a kind of homework. In the past, as you have told me, you have always avoided injections, or even run away from clinics. Because of this, the last thing you remember of these situations is feeling absolutely dreadful, since you have not had the chance to experience that reduction in anxiety I spoke about. [**General description**]

To give you an example, I might ask you, with your consent, to begin by looking at pictures of other people having injections, to move on later to watch others having injections in real life, in one of our clinics here, then to handle needles yourself, before finally trying an injection. The idea is to move from comparatively easy tasks to more difficult ones, at your own pace, always keeping at a level you can just about cope with. That way you get the experience of success, and of anxiety reduction. [**Specific description**]

The idea is that we would work as a team, and I wouldn't force you to take on more than you can handle, all at once. Nevertheless, it would still be my job to keep you moving in the gradual confrontation of the fears. [**Collaborative nature of treatment**]. Of course, there will be times when you will experience considerable discomfort, since you will, after all, be confronting the very things you fear. So, quite a lot of commitment is needed from you, but it often helps to weigh the short-term discomfort of treatment for this fear against the long-term effects of continuing to live a life restricted (and possibly endangered) by it. [**Need for commitment and possibility of discomfort**]

Because it is uncomfortable, and because you'll be working on your own much of the time, I suggest that you might get members of your family to help you with the exercises. Nurse Jones, one of the midwives here, has offered also to talk to you about the treatment and keep an eye on your homework. Also, you are always welcome to observe in the blood test clinic here. [**Need to enlist others**]

This form of treatment is very successful for the majority of our clients, who are able to overcome their fears in a few weeks. [**Likely positive outcome**]. The important thing now is to get started. We'll meet very briefly in two weeks time, to review your progress, and so I suggest we decide on what you'll be doing between now and then to help you achieve your goal of having blood taken and having injections when needed. [**Planning specific relevant tasks**]

COGNITIVELY ORIENTED INTERVENTIONS

General

Cognitive-behavioural clinicians recognize the interactional nature of the physical, cognitive and behavioural systems and therefore aim their interventions at addressing that system where disturbance is most apparent. This intervention may not, however, be direct. For example, in phobias, there is significant autonomic disturbance in the presence of the feared object, yet it is uncommon to attempt to moderate this disturbance by the use of relaxation techniques, since these have generally proved ineffective in phobias.

In the previous section, we saw how cognitive-behaviour therapists use exposure techniques to reduce anxiety through the process of habituation. The cognitive-behaviour therapist recognizes, however, the mediating role of cognitions in determining client behaviour, and thus will use cognitive techniques to maximize the potential of exposure work, and vice versa. A key concept in cognitive-behaviour therapy is the idea of self-efficacy – the client's belief that the results of a particular experience will be positive, and that they have control over those results. In cognitive terms, it is suggested, for example, that exposure exercises, when successful, alter the client's feelings of self-efficacy, change their predictions about future contact with the feared situation and allow learning, through direct experience, that catastrophic predictions do not, in fact, occur. Many cognitive interventions share this characteristic of attempting to alter negative expectations in order to increase client self-efficacy.

The interventions outlined below are all examples of attempts to allow the client to make such alterations, and have now been used quite extensively in the growing field of behavioural medicine, since they are relatively economical of clinician time and address the negative cognitions which often accompany illness (particularly pain states and chronic handicap) directly and effectively. Although it should be stressed that precise selection of particular interventions is rendered easier by accurate assessment, the reader will be able, after reading this section, to offer a number of simple tactics to the client, which are likely to be of value in the more straightforward presentation. Furthermore, it is suggested that the offering of much of this kind of cognitive-behavioural counselling can be integrated into a clinician's style of interaction with clients, rather than being offered as an isolated technique for some individuals. Finally, as with the section on cognitive-behavioural assessment, the following section also represents a way of thinking about client difficulties, which may help the clinician to make appropriate onward referrals in the case of the more complicated client.

Cognitive interventions

There are numerous models of cognitive therapy, all subtly different, and no particular model is described here. However, all the cognitive-behaviour therapies stress the importance of client cognitions in determining behaviour and affect. According to this model, what the client says to himself interacts with experience of the world, so that each influences the other.

In general terms, all cognitive interventions include the following components:

a period of self-monitoring of negative thoughts and other symptoms
a period of skills acquisition, often including debate and practice with the clinician
a period of generalization of the skills learnt into the problem situations, with monitoring and adjustment by the clinician.

Diary-keeping

The client may be asked to keep a diary, noting the occurrence of negative thoughts, e.g.:

I can't cope with this situation
I'll never get well
This pain will go on for ever
I am a useless individual

and also recording events, both positive and negative, between appointments. The diary may include the use of simple rating scales (say 1 to 10) of the severity of particular symptoms (e.g. depressed thoughts, pain, immobility, fatigue) throughout each day.

The diary forms the basis of a tutorial for the client in assessing his/her health status. For example, the clinician may encourage the questioning of particular types of thinking (e.g. generalizing from the particular, catastrophizing, discounting positive aspects) which occur repeatedly, and which are known to be associated with feelings of low self-efficacy and with low mood. The clinician may also note the occurrence of positive events, draw these to the attention of the client and offer appropriate reinforcement for task achievement.

Challenging negative thoughts

The clinician, perhaps using diary material, encourages the client to generate 'coping thoughts' based on a more realistic appraisal of his/her situation, e.g.:

This situation is difficult, but I have managed before
I've felt more ill than this, but recovered
I have had pain before and it has passed or decreased
I am having difficulties with this problem, but am competent at other things.

Calibrating discomfort levels

As part of the challenging process, the client is asked to use a pain (or discomfort, fatigue, difficulty, etc.) thermometer, to measure particular instances of difficulty against earlier occurrences. The client therefore learns to set the difficulty in context and thereby experiences increased control.

Self-reward

The client is asked to identify particular activities or objects which s/he values, and voluntarily to restrict access to these to situations where his/her desired goals have been met. Self-reward can also be covert – the client is asked to ensure that s/he congratulates her/himself after each occurrence of coping (e.g. climbing a flight of stairs). As part of the process, the client may also be asked to refuse inappropriate rewards from others – for example, expressions of concern or reassurance, or the performance of tasks on behalf of the client. The client should thus learn to distinguish between those behaviours which increase and decrease handicap.

Scheduling

Usually combined with self-reward, this involves the client in contracting with the clinician to perform a schedule of mutually agreed tasks of gradually increasing difficulty. The process shares features with exposure advice, since the client may well experience anxiety reduction and changes in negative expectations (e.g. about the likelihood of pain occurring following task performance). Scheduling should be so negotiated that the client experiences the maximum reward for the minimum effort in the early stages, thus enhancing feelings of control and increasing the likelihood of compliance with later, and possibly more difficult, tasks.

Distraction/relaxation

Although these techniques have fallen into disuse in the treatment of focal anxiety, many clients with pain syndromes find them of use, probably because of the increase in feelings of control of the symptoms. By contrast, some clients find that deliberate focusing on the pain, imagining it rising and falling, brings relief, possibly by decreasing the level of anxiety associated with the pain, through habituation.

PROGRESS CHECKLIST 4

Cognitively-oriented interventions

> self-monitoring of negative thoughts and other symptoms
> skills acquisition, often including debate and practice with the clinician
> generalization of the skills learnt into the problem situations, with monitoring by the clinician
> diary-keeping – thoughts, events – use as tutorial
> challenging negative thoughts
> calibrating discomfort levels
> self-reward – activities, objects – ignoring inappropriate rewards
> scheduling – gradual increases in activities
> distraction/relaxation – pain focusing

Throughout the process, the emphasis is on the client learning to test and use these techniques in real life. In the example given below, a client has avoided activity for a long period after a severe chest infection. He describes continuing breathlessness, associated chest pain on exertion, and extreme fatigue following exertion. He is currently spending twenty hours per day in bed, and avoiding work and domestic duties. There is no evidence of enduring physical damage. Here, he discusses with his GP the first steps in their agreed programme of gradually increasing activity and tuition in a variety of coping tactics. The GP begins by discussing his diary-keeping. She goes on to check a series of tasks they have discussed, and draws the client's attention to non-coping thinking, elicits alternative coping thoughts and checks possible pitfalls during future tasks.

PRACTICAL EXAMPLE 3

Post-viral fatigue

GP: So, Mr Robinson, looking at your diaries, it seems like most exertion leads to you feeling absolutely exhausted?

Client: That's right.

GP: Yet there are some things you're still able to do? [**Encouraging challenging**]

Client: Well, for example, I can drive for about twenty minutes, and I can manage to walk round the library.

GP: So the thought you described about being *unable* to do anything at all is a bit of an overstatement? [**Identifying non-coping thinking style**] Is there some more coping thought you could put in its place? [**Encouraging identification of strengths**]

Client: I could say 'Even though it's difficult, I managed to get out today'.

GP: Excellent. You might add: 'And the tiredness was not as bad as yesterday'. [**Encouraging calibration**]

Client: That's right.

GP: Now tell me what you're going to do this week to improve your performance? [**Contracting scheduling of activities**]

Client: I'm going to stay out of bed for six hours each day, and I also want to walk for twenty minutes each day.

GP: That sounds great. I think that will be very tiring. How will you cope? [**Checking availability of coping tactics**]

Client: I'll remind myself of last year, when I had to work all night, several nights running to meet a client's deadline, but I still got through it all right. [**Calibration**] I'll think of the bath I'm going to enjoy when I get home. [**Self-reward**]

GP: Yes, I think that's quite excellent. Have you got a fall-back position if that's too much? [**Trying to ensure success**]

Client: Hmmm. Yes, I could aim for just ten minutes of walking each day.

CONCLUSION

In summary, cognitive-behavioural interventions present the clinician with a series of relatively simple tactics for addressing a variety of client difficulties. Although cognitive-behavioural therapy was originally used chiefly with anxiety disorders, and the anxiety component of many medical complaints has been stressed above, the clinician will readily see the applicability of these formulations to an increasing range of complaints as familiarity with the behavioural model grows.

Often, the person wishing to employ such interventions is deterred by the seeming complexity of the assessment process, and by its apparently time-consuming nature. However, it has been emphasized throughout that much of the actual therapeutic work is done by clients themselves, in the form of self-treatment, whilst time spent on the initial assessment will be repaid, given the high degree of effectiveness associated with cognitive-behavioural interventions, by decreased consultation time in the following months and even years.

This chapter should provide sufficient general guidelines to use such interventions as part of everyday consultations. The important thing is to integrate cognitive-behavioural interventions into one's clinical style in daily interactions with clients, and this comes most readily through regular practice. Cognitive-behavioural interviewing is a highly focal and directive style, which some clinicians initially find unfamiliar, but which clients respond to extremely positively.

SUGGESTED FURTHER READING

Hawton, K., Salkovskis, P.M., Kirk, J. and Clark, D.M. (1989) *Cognitive Behaviour Therapy for Psychiatric Problems: A Practical Guide*, Oxford: Oxford University Press.

Marks, I.M. (1987) *Behavioural Psychotherapy: The Maudsley Handbook of Clinical Administration*, London: Wright.

Turk, D.C., Meichenbaum, D. and Genest, M. (1983) *Pain and Behavioural Medicine. A Cognitive-behavioural Perspective*, New York: Guilford Press.

Part III

The role of the doctor and other professionals

Chapter 14

Looking after yourself

Roger Higgs

The skills of self-care start with a paradox. Any of us who work in professions related to health or social care should be experts (or be training ourselves to be experts) in how to look after people. At this point in human history (and in the reading of this book!) no one should be in any doubt that competence in the purely technical areas of our work may be hard to acquire but it is not enough. We have to understand, be able to care for and organize care for these people who put their trust in our professional hands. As experts in the field, we should be able to apply those same ideas to ourselves. What is more, failure to do so might be thought to undermine our professional work or status. What professional footballer would listen to a manager who drank so heavily he was manifestly unfit? How could he do his work, or continue to be respected? And yet in the field of health care, this does not seem to hold. Outsiders would say that few of us appear to pay much attention to our own needs and care for ourselves well. Little is written about this, and few studies have been made of self care for the health professional. But the impression of doctors, nurses and social workers risking their physical, psychological and social health is apparent everywhere. Why should this be, and what should be done?

Let us look first at an example. When as a school leaver I first began to think of becoming a doctor, I took a temporary holiday job as a theatre porter in our local hospital. On my second day I was assigned to the chest surgeon's list, and noted that he was operating that morning on two patients with lung cancer. To my surprise I met the surgeon on his way into theatre, stubbing out his cigarette on the sole of his shoe. During a lull in proceedings from behind the anonymity of my mask I asked, in as careful a way as I could, how he could reconcile this work with continuing to smoke. The subsequent explosion could be imagined! I learned a great deal at that moment about the medical power structure, but the different comments of those colleagues who were still prepared to talk to me did give me some insight into the way professionals view themselves or each other. 'That surgeon thinks he is different, in some way, from the rest of us.' 'It's his own business isn't it? If he gets cancer, serves him right for giving himself airs.' 'I expect he thinks it can't happen to him.' 'But he's OK – the scientific evidence isn't *absolutely* watertight, and smoking doesn't always cause lung cancer.' 'It's the work. I know I smoke too but I certainly couldn't get my work done without it.' 'The pressure is too much: how do they expect us to get by without?' 'I expect it helps him to sympathize with patients in the clinic.' 'He knows all about it anyway.'

Smoking habits among health professionals, especially doctors, have changed radically since then, and I only intend to focus on the issue of a smoking doctor here in as much as it symbolizes something about attitudes that we take to our work. The important issues that need to be examined are the assumptions that we make about ourselves as professionals, our role and status and the values we espouse when it comes to thinking about ourselves and acting upon it. Each of the comments which were made about the surgeon say something about these ideas and will help us to focus on how we might be better at looking after ourselves than the previous generation.

'WE'RE DIFFERENT' – ASPECTS OF BELONGING TO A PROFESSION

Few of us get past the moments when we first set foot on the wards as students or finally qualify without feeling a strong emotion. It's exhilarating – we're there at last; or terrifying – am I really up to it? There is some sense in which we are marked out now as different. 'Don't ever change', said a good friend when she heard I wanted to read medicine – yet clearly I would. She meant (I think!) that I should try to preserve that human, approachable side of my character or behaviour; but it really said a lot about how remote she felt that doctors as people were when they were acting in their professional role. That phrase actually encapsulated the prime difficulty of professional life: the ability to view oneself as different, in terms of duties, responsibilities and skills, but the same in terms of human make-up, needs and capacities. It is this very tension that provides the necessity for some aspects of professional behaviour.

One of the first requirements of a professional is probably some form of detachment. Our normal human reactions to a stinking wound, or a frighteningly disturbed individual, or someone with no home to go to, do have to be subjected to some form of control, or the work couldn't be done. We learn by modelling on our colleagues, by precept and sometimes through trial and error, what is the correct distance to keep between our professional self and our personal self, between the feelings and their expression in words or action, between care and friendship, between empathy and personal involvement. We do this in order to present some form of consistency and in acknowledgement of the legitimate demands of the next client or patient, and the one after that: we cannot risk becoming completely involved in one 'case', as we might if that 'case' were a friend, a lover or our child.

Yet we cannot risk either being too detached that we offer nothing of ourselves. Studies of patient satisfaction, placebo reaction, the nursing process or social case-work all show that to be effective the individual professional must invest *something* of herself in the work. Without this, efforts may be less effective and we risk at a deeper level a dangerous splitting of our emotional responses. But this boundary, the judgement of the correct distance between ourselves and those we are trying to help, is itself a most important area for care, for checking and reassessment throughout our professional life. We must attend to it regularly while we follow our vocation.

'IT'S OUR WORK': THE LIMITS OF VOCATION AND MOTIVATION

It is intrinsic to the idea of vocation that there is something about the work we do that is more than 'just a job'. This causes incidents that many of us will recognize as we struggle with the balance between ourselves as individuals who stop work at the end of the day and as professionals who remain constantly on duty. Though it would be wrong to think that many other workers don't become involved with and identified with their work in a deep way, there is a sense that society expects health workers to retain their professional skills and their readiness to act off duty as well as on ('Is there an architect in the house?' is an unusual cry). In many primitive societies, healers go through an instruction initiation period which sets them apart (like the Shona healers, who are considered locally to 'spend three years underwater with the mermaids'): they are considered to be in touch with the divine when they return to normal society. In Western societies we can still trace elements of this at work in our training systems, but we should be alert to the dangers, whether it is a full blown 'God complex' that seems to afflict some prima donnas in the health services, or the very understandable conflict between person and role – which most of us find difficult to disentangle when a family member becomes ill. We have a duty to provide care. Assumption of this vocation, without careful reflection however, may lead us to several unwise conclusions. Like everyone else, we should put limits to the amount and length of the work that we do, and realize that as people we are not immune to the ordinary afflictions of those around us, like fatigue or illness. Family and social relations need to be kept in good order.

One of the things that you're traditionally not supposed to say when you go for an interview for health care training is 'I want to do it to help people'. Nevertheless, this simple line is part of many people's motivation. This is just as well, because the demands made by most work in the caring professions do assume a fair measure of altruism. Values about life, welfare and relationships are in some senses shared in common and are intrinsic to the way in which the work is done. We should not expect to leave a clinical task halfway through because it is 5 pm and our evening off, and it comes as an amazing shock when someone challenges that view. An African medical missionary described borrowing a chief's Land Rover to provide the lights to do an emergency operation outdoors at night, and was halfway through with the belly open when the car was required and driven off!

Nearer home, there is a great difference of opinion as to whether and when strike action is justified to press a claim or a protest. The imperative is to help others, and the law as well as professional bodies see us as having a clear duty to care and provide care for those entrusted to us. But this has to have limits, both in a practical and a moral sense. We cannot help everybody, so there is a sort of 'moral triage' which we have to learn to engage in in our heads when we begin a busy job: how to maximize our effectiveness. How to make best use of our time in many ways is an ethical issue no less important to review than the use of any other scarce resource. It involves a delicate moral balance between helping others, reducing suffering and avoiding harm to ourselves and those to whom we have personal duties. Few thoughtful professionals will not be caught one day in the conflict between family and work, or spending a lot of time on one task and having to skimp another. It is the stuff of which great dramas are made and may require deep and prolonged thought. But it also has ordinary everyday consequences for avoiding inefficient use of time, like consciously working towards making ourselves efficient in non-clinical areas (like paperwork) as well as the immediate professional tasks. It is surprising how many professionals still pride themselves on 'being hopeless at all these things', as if writing reports and being polite to people were for 'mere mortals'.

'THE WORK MUST BE DONE': QUALITY AND COST

None of us doubts that we have chosen to do what we do because it is so important, yet we can be deceived by the very importance of our work into several errors, which may lead to personal damage. One is that if work is good, more work must be better. 'How are you, doc? Busy I suppose' is the refrain. We are busy, but addiction to this busy-ness can become a subtle but very destructive dependency. It may blind us to assessing the quality, and not just the quantity of our work, or to feeling that in every situation we are called to 'do something': no one likes to be seen to be unhelpful. Maybe future generations will see doctors' tranquillizer prescribing this way in years to come. It may prevent us seeing what happens to our family and social life when our work *always* takes precedence. It may stop us asking what the work is for, or may entrap us in a cynical career folly where the results of the work, where it gets *us* to, become more important than what the work actually is, what it does for the people we work for or with. Broken medical and nursing marriages and partnerships bear witness to poor judgements here: and the effects of the alternative dependencies of drugs or drink on stressed professionals are a regular feature of reports to professional bodies.

The demands of the work may make the worker vulnerable not only to her own idealism but also to exploitation from others. Being exploited by colleagues may be more easy to see than being exploited by an institution. Here partners, employers, management groups or governments may put unreasonable pressure on young and enthusiastic colleagues, with disastrous consequences. This 'scorched-earth' approach to professional training is still sadly prevalent. We are in it, and in one sense have only ourselves to blame. We owe the duty to care: but not at every cost in all circumstances. We also owe a duty to care for ourselves and those we work with.

'IT CAN'T HAPPEN TO ME': RISKS AND RULES

When we're young it's important to take risks: and mature risk-taking has to be part of every professional's style. Somehow, the confidence that we can be beavering away in an epidemic or a social disaster area without it affecting us is a necessary defence against the fear that we all feel when confronted by disaster. Perhaps acknowledging that fear would be a good road to health – we shall return to that theme. But reasonable precautions remain reasonable precautions, for ourselves and those we care for. The nurse who lifts a heavy patient without help, the phlebotomist who takes blood without a hepatitis B immunization, the social worker who sees a violent client alone, are all declaring 'I'm different – it can't happen to me'. They may be right. But it could. That things don't very often go wrong may be due to our knowledge and skills, or that we are younger, fitter and better nourished than many of those we serve. But there is no excuse for taking undue physical or psychological risks with ourselves. Doctors and nurses commonly ignore disease, and then when they are ill panic and assume that it is a very complicated or difficult medical problem. Routine arrangements and checks are ignored: many don't get registered with a general practitioner, they self-treat or are looked after informally by colleagues or family. Sometimes this results in their being managed physically at an inappropriately high level by colleagues who may have forgotten their ordinary skills or who want to be kind or make short cuts.

> A casualty officer had a sore throat. Acting quite against what he would normally advise and without seeking advice from his GP he took Ampicillin. A florid rash appeared, and he was unacceptable in casualty on aesthetic as well as health grounds. As the diagnosis was in doubt all sorts of dire infectious possibilities were raised which threatened the closure of casualty before the physician on call pointed out that this rash was specific for someone with glandular fever who was incorrectly prescribed Ampicillin.

> A nurse and her two-year-old child went to stay with the grandmother, who was a senior medical academic. The child became ill during the stay and was admitted by a consultant friend of the grandmother to his own ward with a diagnosis of pneumonia. As a favour the usual admitting procedures were bypassed, and no lumbar puncture was done. The child had meningitis which went undiagnosed and incorrectly treated for several days.

The rules in professional health care are easy to state. If it's important for my patients, it's important for me. If it's not important for them, whatever am I doing it for? Prevention is no less important for professionals than for patients or clients. Each person should have his own health adviser, if possible, separate and confidential from immediate colleagues and management. Families have a right to appropriate health care too. Where psychological or employment issues become of greater importance, independent assessment can become crucial. A GP who had a drinking and marriage problem changed partnerships and unwisely followed the pattern of the partnership he joined and became the patient of one of his partners, as did his wife. All went well until he began to feel under strain, when he began to drink and to prescribe valium for himself. When the drinking was suspected by his partners, his previous notes were available for them, and a very messy situation developed in which no one acted well, and no one had the support or professional help they deserved.

'THE PRESSURE IS TOO MUCH': STRESS AND PROFESSIONAL LIFE

For many reasons, some of which we've glanced at, the helping professionals can easily be caught in their own machine, and work longer or more intensively than is healthy. Probably the entry to most professions involves in some senses a 'baptism of fire' for junior members. At worst, this ensures the survival of the fittest. Emotional stability, or a thick hide, is bought by the group at the high price of reduced sensitivity. Cynically, it sometimes seems as if older members who survive will be determined not to get caught a second time; or else they believe that what they went through was in some senses a necessary professional initiation. That may well be, in some cases, but even if the idea is challenged, and work pressures distributed in what may appear to be a more equitable way, there still remains a central issue: however much we may gain satisfaction from our work, helping other people is intrinsically stressful. Few of us will end up working routinely with the kind of people with whom we have grown up or with problems to which we have become accustomed from childhood. We shall have to deal with illness, death, madness or poverty to a degree that we have seldom previously experienced. Since the aim of our professions is to prevent, avoid, or change such things – even that they are to be fought or opposed – we may have personal difficulty coming to terms with them in our own lives. Unless we had a remarkable upbringing, it is unlikely that we have previously integrated within ourselves the threats that they might pose to us personally. The central preoccupation of our work is with something that society otherwise thinks of as bad. Instead of repressing thought about it, or shunning it as others may, we have to face it head on. It's probably time we realized that this can be a very tough assignment.

Most of us cope by a variety of mechanisms. Assuming, as we've said, that 'it couldn't happen to us' we make the client or patient 'them', and different from us as a class as well as individuals. It's difficult when the two classes coincide as we've seen: when nurse becomes patient, social worker becomes client. 'Oh you're a doctor. I'm so sorry', said the physician who was examining me, and immediately (and for the first time!) looked me in the face – but stopped examining me forthwith and began to tell me about his problems! We develop jargon – looking after people who are dying becomes 'terminal care' and so on. We resort to the technical, and avoid the emotional. We must have jokes, with fellow professionals, which are extremely funny (unless you're a lay person from outside). We keep our distance emotionally, as we have seen, but physically as well. A medical student learning massage said how wonderful it was at last to begin to touch people in a real way again. We keep our strong emotions to ourselves, if we can. And so on. But sooner or later, comes the crunch. Stresses that have been tucked away may resurface or habits may become inappropriate.

> A young paediatrician who had been horrified by several cases of child sexual abuse, and had not been able to share this with a senior member or discuss this with anyone, was threatened by a potential rapist during her work. Although nothing came of this and she was quickly rescued, she was unable to return to work for many weeks and required intensive therapy, in which the feelings of what she had previously witnessed emerged and could begin to be integrated.

THE NEED FOR SUPERVISION AND SUPPORT

Communicating and relating well with patients or clients is at the heart of all professional work, and many professionals find that as the work leaves the technical area and approaches personal human issues it changes. It may become more rewarding, or more difficult. Surprisingly, it probably becomes more stressful and more demanding. It is tempting to think that in this more 'natural' area of our work we can be more relaxed and will need less help. The reverse may well be the case. Our own untutored or unreflective reasons may well be inappropriate to the matter in hand. Some are good at making these judgements, others are not.

We may not be able to tell without reflection. The newer professions of counselling and psychoanalysis and some of the personal social services insist that early professional experience is always accompanied by detailed supervision. Some people continue to be supervised all their lives. The extraordinary thing about the health and some social care services is that not only is no requirement or provision made for supervision, but that it is positively discouraged. Even in a straightforward educational model, this is somewhat primitive. Teaching is seen as a transmission of knowledge and skills: in the primitive model, feedback and reassessment are not considered a priority, so in the pressure of work a professional depends on her own introspection, or an unexpected outcome, to tell her how she is working. It is clear from reactions both of the public and of governments that this must change. Audit and evaluation must be part of every professional life, and must be built in to the practice, not an optional extra. In this way it can become a way of handling stress, rather than creating further pressures.

Where stressful events clearly occur, however, health care professions are slowly waking up to the realization that more is required. The best in general practitioner training now offers personal supervision in a straightforward professional sense to the learner, and group supervision and support from peers with an experienced group leader. In many cases, young practitioners have continued to meet to discuss the issues that cause stress and anxiety. Many nursing teams in personally challenging jobs, like intensive paediatric care or terminal illness, have regular access to an outside counsellor or to team support meetings. That these activities are still not seen as routine and necessary in spite of their proven value is a monument to the 'if you can't stand the heat get out of the kitchen' school of professional training. Now that the kitchen work is complex and expensive, and new workers scarce, it is possible that the human costs of not providing support and supervision, especially at the time of training, may become obvious to those who plan services. What supervision will be given in a job may be as important a question as the time off and pay.

'BUT I'M OK'

Successful and skilful professionals may well be able to see and steer round many of these traps. You, the reader, may be feeling that the difficulties are exaggerated. You're enjoying your job, you're doing well, what's the problem? This chapter certainly is not motivated by some principle of pessimism. Although there is a welcome atmosphere of questioning and reassessment in Western society about the benefits of health care and welfare, how it should be delivered and the priorities that should be used, the author of this chapter (while having strong views in these debates also!) is not questioning the value of the work that professionals do: quite the reverse. The point is that it is seldom made explicit that most types of activity do have side-effects and risks. Recently society has been made much more aware of the risks of, say, powerful paternalistic doctoring or expensive welfare agencies, and as a result traditional attitudes and rewards are being challenged. But what has not been adequately assessed or expressed is what the side-effects and risks are to the professional as a *person*. While financial or emotional rewards remain high, these risks will be accepted without question. But this is hardly healthy for those whose job it is to help others look at the risks they face: and may be unacceptable if the rewards begin to lose their value. If we think what we do is valuable or even vital for society we also owe it to society to keep our profession and its practice in good shape.

Sometimes it is this very refusal of the professional to acknowledge that there are problems which require attention that creates difficulty in relationships between the profession and the rest of society. If standards are high, that is fine, but if ranks close when there is a criticism, or if the professional refuses to acknowledge that a mistake has been made, or that professional responses could be improved in some way, then a credibility gap emerges between professions and the rest of society, and between individual professionals and their clients. There is a paradox here that this chapter will not resolve. The public expects professional skill of the highest, but personal approachability and openness also, and this may imply some evidence of weakness or vulnerability. Feet of clay are not an exception but the rule. Some have seen the greatest power for the healer to be when the healer herself is in some senses 'wounded'. Certainly realizing that the healer has needs which may be greater than the patient's is a theme of great importance in psychoanalytic writing. Whether this is accepted or not, the 'perfect' professional in doing her best will realize that in the real world what is done can never be absolutely perfect and she should be open about this: she also has an understanding of her own potential fallibility and human failings. Perceptive outsiders realize that professionals are never so dangerous as when they think they are perfectly safe and can do nothing wrong. The history of litigation against professionals bears witness not just to professional failings but to professionals failing to perceive these failings. Being 'holier than thou' invites 'thou' to put it to the test.

Litigation may bring us down with a bump and remind us that there is a practical job to do where things may go right or wrong, and that looking after ourselves is a practical skill with outcomes. The professional emerging from the teaching institution where rules of action can be made to apply may find herself in practice having to think on her feet, faced by problems in a shape not encountered before. The new professional must be prepared to face this uncertainty. She must examine ideals in the light of new realities, and be prepared to take on during a professional lifetime new knowledge and skills, and re-examine old attitudes. Learning from life is a slogan which enables the professional to face practical challenges by being a self-directed and self-motivated learner constantly assessing and updating what is required of her.

Assessing oneself may be easy if things go badly wrong, but most of us will make sure they don't and so we need a method where it can be built into our professional practice. Some professions have regular peer review structure, job reviews from managers or feedback systems from colleagues or clients. In their absence, three suggestions are made:

1   The professional should regularly record (with permission) her interactions with patients/clients either on audio or videotape and ask a colleague to join in assessing them. With the right approach this can be invaluable.
2   Second, any strong emotion in professional encounters, whether it is anger, fear, love or disdain, is a signal for reflective examination. It may be that there is a moral issue that has not been identified, or it may be a clash between what the profession demands and the person feels able to give.
3   Lastly, we do not stop developing as people or professionals throughout our lives, so if we are to pay attention to that we will sometimes need help at difficult points. Friends,

colleagues and family will be invaluable, but sometimes it is helpful to have personal or group support.

Pacing oneself, looking at motivation, being true to oneself where there is an incongruity with what work demands, identifying and providing new skills with new challenges – all these may be hard to initiate without someone else holding a mirror to our life from time to time. Looking after yourself starts with looking *at* yourself. That can be tough, but what comes after may well be easier.

SUGGESTED FURTHER READING

Bennet, G. (1979) *Patients and their Doctors*, London: Ballière Tindal.
Campbell, A. (1984) *Moderated Love*, London: SPCK.
Campbell, A. and Higgs, H. (1982) *In that Case*, London: Darton Longman and Todd.
Gillon, R. (1985) *Philosophical Medical Ethics*, London: Wiley.
Schon, D.A. (1987) *Educating the Reflective Practitioner*, San Francisco: Jossey-Bass.

Chapter 15

The role of other organizations

Roslyn Corney

There are a number of organizations and agencies specifically set up to deal with the psycho-social problems of patients and it is important that the doctor is aware of this and refers on for extra help where necessary. One team or ward may have the capacity for plenty of this type of work and can manage relatively demanding cases, while another team will only be able to cope with basic work and will need to refer many cases on.

A small proportion of general hospital patients will clearly have to be referred to the psychiatric services. These people may have lost emotional control or are disabled psychologically, they may exhibit bizarre behaviour or experience intense emotions. However, there will be another larger group of disturbed patients who do not need to be referred to the psychiatric services. People in this group may have coped with their problems when well but the experience of being ill has brought about some sort of crisis.

Within the hospital, social workers, psychologists, counsellors (including nurse counsellors) and nursing staff can be called upon to help. Other professionals include physiotherapists and occupational therapists. Home care staff including general practitioners, health visitors, district nurses, community psychiatric nurses and social workers may help at discharge. If these professionals are unable to help directly they may be aware of local facilities which may benefit the patient and his family.

Another important resource is other patients. Individuals may gain most benefit by talking to someone else who has had the illness, operation or experience. These individuals may still be on the hospital ward but if not, patients are often willing to come back and talk to other patients. Self-help groups are numerous and can be extremely helpful and supportive.

Many national organizations and charities have local groups and branches all over England, Scotland, Wales and Northern Ireland. A useful resource directory has been compiled by the Mental Health Foundation, *Someone to Talk to Directory 1985*, published by Routledge.

Addresses of a number of national organizations are given below. Details of local offices can be obtained from the central office of that particular organization.

ADDICTION

Alanon
Family Groups UK and Eire
61 Great Dover Street
London SE1 4YF
Tel: 071 403 0888
(Help and advice for those with alcohol problems)

Alcoholics Anonymous
General Service Office
P.O. Box 1
Stonebow House
York YO1 2NJ
Tel: 0904 644026
(Help and advice for those with alcohol problems)

ASH
5–11 Mortimer Street
London W1N 7RH
Tel: 071 637 9843
(Help, advice and information to give up smoking)

Gamblers Anonymous
17–23 Blantyre Street
Cheyne Walk
London SW10
Tel: 071 352 3060
(Help, advice and information with disability)

Parents Anonymous
7 Park Grove off Broadway
Worseley
Walden
Greater Manchester
Tel: 061 790 6544
(A support group for parents of drug users)

Release
169 Commercial Street
London E1 6BW
Tel: 071 603 8654 / 071 377 5905
(Initial counselling on drug use and referral. Advice on law, women's rights, abortion, etc.)

BEREAVEMENT COUNSELLING

Compassionate Friends
50 Woodwaye
Watford
Hertfordshire
Tel: 0923 23279
(An international organization of bereaved parents. Offers advice, support to parents who lose a child)

Cruse (National Organisation for the Widowed and their Children)
Cruse House
126 Sheen Road
Richmond
Surrey TW9 1VR
Tel: 081 940 4818
(Support for widowed and their children)

National Still-Birth Study Group
66 Harley Street
London W1N 1AE
(Help, advice and information)

CANCER SUPPORT

BACUP (British Association of Cancer United Patients)
121 Charterhouse Street
London EC1M 6AA
Tel: 071 608 1661 (Information Service)
071 608 1038 (Counselling Service)
(Help, information and counselling for cancer patients and their families)

National Society for Cancer Relief
Michael Sobell House
30 Dorset Square
London NW1
Tel: 071 402 8125
(Funds networks of terminal-care units and makes block grants or allowances)

COUNSELLING SERVICES

British Association of Counselling
37a Sheep Street
Rugby
Warwickshire CV21 3BX
Tel: 0788 78328
(A national body which can provide information about local counselling services and individual counsellors)

Family Service Units
207 Old Marylebone Road
London NW1 5QP
Tel: 071 402 5175
(To prevent the breakdown of family and community life by providing services)

Family Welfare Association
501–505 Kingsland Road
London E8 4AU
Tel: 071 245 6251
(Help, advice and information for families)

National Association of Young People's Counselling and Advisory Services
Teenage Information Network
102 Harper Road
London SE1 6AQ
Tel: 071 403 2444
(Counselling, advice and activities for young people)

Samaritans
46 Marshall Street
London W1V 1LR
Tel: 071 439 2224
(Telephone service for the distressed and suicidal. Befriending service)

Westminster Pastoral Foundation
23 Kensington Square
London W8 5HN
Tel: 071 937 6956
(To provide a national counselling service, open to all in need of help)

DISABILITY

British Red Cross Society
9 Grosvenor Crescent
London SW1X 7EJ
Tel: 071 235 5454
(Community welfare services for the disabled)

Crossroad Care Attendant Scheme Trust
94a Cotton Road
Rugby
Warwickshire CV21 4LN
Tel: 0788 61536
(Provides care and support to the disabled, help for parents, families and friends)

Disabled Living Foundation
380–384 Harrow Road
London W9 2HU
Tel: 071 289 6111
(Provides an aids centre, information service and publications)

Invalid Children's Aid Association
Unit 151
Stratford Workshops
Burford Road
London E15
Tel: 081 519 5266
(Help and advice for parents with handicapped children)

National Association for Deaf/Blind and Rubella Handicap
311 Grays Inn Road
London WC1X 8PT
Tel: 071 278 1005
(Concerned with children and adults who are handicapped as a result of congenital rubella)

National Deaf Children's Society
45 Hereford Road
London W2 5AH
Tel: 071 387 8033
(Represents deaf children's interests nationally and locally through a large network of self-help groups)

Royal National Institute for the Blind
224 Great Portland Street
London W1N 6AA
Tel: 071 388 1266
(Help, advice and information. List of schools available on request)

Royal National Institute for the Deaf
105 Gower Street
London WC1E 6AH
Tel: 071 387 8033
(The main umbrella organization representing the deaf)

Spastics Society
12 Park Crescent
London W1N 4EQ
Tel: 071 636 5020
(The care, treatment, education and training of spastics. Help, advice, support and information services)

SPOD Committee on Sexual and Personal Relationships of the Disabled
Brook House
2–16 Torrington Place
London WC1
Tel: 071 637 4712
(Promotes awareness of the problems and factual information and advice to the disabled)

DIVORCE ADVICE

National Council for the Divorced and Separated
13 High Street
Little Shelford
Cambridge CB2 5ES
(Help, advice and information)

GENERAL ADVICE

National Association of Citizens Advice Bureaux
115–123 Pentonville Road
London N1 9LZ
Tel: 071 833 2181

MARRIAGE COUNSELLING

National Marriage Guidance Council (Relate)
Herbert Gray College
Little Church Street
Rugby
Warwickshire CV21 3AP
Tel: 0788 73241
(Appointments and counselling for married and single people in need of counselling)

MEDICAL DISORDERS

British Heart Foundation
102 Gloucester Place
London W1H 4DH
Tel: 071 935 0185
(Help, advice and information)

Chest, Heart and Stroke Association
123 Whitecross Street
London EC1
Tel: 071 490 7999
(Support for those suffering from a stroke, chest or heart disease)

MENTAL ILLNESS AND HANDICAP

Alzheimer's Disease Society
Bank Lodges
158–160 Balham High Road
London SW12
Tel: 081 675 6557
(To give support and practical help to families where there is Alzheimer's disease)

MENCAP
117–123 Golden Lane
London EC1Y 0RT
Tel: 071 253 9433
(Organization concerning both adults and children who are mentally handicapped)

MIND (National Association for Mental Health)
22 Harley Street
London W1N 2ED
Tel: 071 637 0741
(A service concerning all aspects of mental health, legal, counselling and a pressure group)

National Schizophrenia Fellowship
78–79 Victoria Road
Surbiton
Surrey KT6 4NS
Tel: 081 390 3651
(Help and support for sufferers and their families)

OLD AGE AND DISABILITY

Age Concern
Bernard Sunley House
60 Pitcairn Road
Mitcham
Surrey CR4 3LL
Tel: 081 640 5431
(A clearing house for information on all aspects of help for senior citizens)

PREGNANCY AND THE FAMILY

Association for Post-Natal Illness
7 Gowan Avenue
London SW6
Tel: 071 731 4867
(A nationwide telephone support scheme for those with post-natal depression, promotes research)

British Pregnancy Advisory Service
7 Belgrave Road
London SW1V 1QB
Tel: 071 222 0985
(Help and advice on problems arising from pregnancy, also advice on male and female sterilization)

Childline
Faraday Building
Addle Hill
London EC4
Tel: 071 236 2380
(Advice for children at risk of abuse)

Miscarriage Support Group
Alexandra House
Oldham Terrace
London W3
Tel: 081 992 8637
(Support and help for women and families who have had a miscarriage)

National Childbirth Trust
9 Queensborough Terrace
London W2 3TB
Tel: 071 221 3833
(Services include ante-natal classes for mothers, post-natal support, education work in schools)

National Society for the Prevention of Cruelty to Children
Headquarters National
67 Saffron Hill
London EC1
Tel: 071 242 1626
(Help, advice and information)

Parents Anonymous
6–9 Manor Gardens
London N7 6LA
Tel: 071 263 8918
(To offer friendship and help to those parents who are tempted to abuse their child)

SEXUALITY COUNSELLING

AIDS – Terrence Higgins Trust
PO Box No. BM AIDS
London WC1N 3XX
Tel: 071 833 2971
(Provides support, aid and information to AIDS sufferers and their families)

Albany Trust, The
24 Chester Square
London SW1 9HF
Tel: 071 730 5871
(Offers advice to homosexuals and lesbians)

London Gay Switchboard
BM Switchboard
London WC1N 3XX
Tel: 071 837 7324
(24 hrs telephone support service for gay men and women, information legal/medical referrals, accommodation service)

VICTIM SUPPORT AND RAPE

National Association of Victim Support Schemes
Cranmer House
39 Brixton Road
London SW9
Tel: 071 735 9166
(To provide information, support and practical help to people who have suffered as a result of crime)

Rape Crisis Centre
P.O. Box 69
London WC1X 9NJ
Tel: 071 837 1600
(A central counselling service for all women who have been raped or sexually assaulted)

Index